MW01254069

Innovations in Community Mental Health

Edited by
Saul Cooper, MA
and
Timothy H. Lentner, MSW

Professional Resource Press
Sarasota, Florida

Published by Professional Resource Press
(An imprint of Professional Resource Exchange, Inc.)
Post Office Box 15560
Sarasota, FL 34277-1560

The copy editor for this book was Patricia Hammond, the managing editor was Debbie Fink, the production coordinator was Laurie Girsch, and the cover designer was Jami Stinnet.

Library of Congress Cataloging-in-Publication Data

Innovations in community mental health / edited by Saul Cooper and
    Timothy H. Lentner.
        p.   cm.
    Includes bibliographical references.
    ISBN 0-943158-76-1 (paperbound ed.)
    1. Community mental health services--United States. 2. Community
mental health services--United States--Administration. I. Lentner,
Timothy H., date.
RA790.6.I53   1992
362.2'2'0973--dc20   92-5819
                                                          CIP

Dedication

This book is dedicated to all those Mental Health professionals who have toiled for the past couple of decades with skill, flexibility, and an unquenching commitment to those of our clients with physical and/or psychological problems, in an attempt to assure them a decent quality of life regardless of the nature of their problems.

List of Contributors

Anthony Broskowski, PhD, Director of Health Care Research and Evaluation of the Prudential Insurance Company, Roseland, NJ.

Saul Cooper, MA, Director, Washtenaw County, Human Services Department, Ann Arbor, MI, and Adjunct Associate Professor of Psychology, University of Michigan, Ann Arbor, MI.

David L. Cutler, MD, Professor of Psychiatry and Director of the Public Psychiatry Training Program, Department of Psychiatry, Oregon Health Sciences University, Portland, OR.

Morris L. Eaddy, PhD, President and Chief Executive Officer of Lakeview Center, Inc., Pensacola, FL.

James O. Gibson, Chairman of GibsonFisher Ltd., Columbus, OH.

Loretta K. Haggard, is presently working on joint JD/MSW degree at Washington University, St. Louis, MO.

David S. Hargrove, PhD, Professor and Chair, Department of Psychology, University of Mississippi, University, MS.

Gerald Landsberg, DSW, MPA, Chairman of the Social Welfare Programs and Policies at the New York University Graduate School of Social Work, New York, NY.

Timothy H. Lentner, MSW, Program Administrator, Adult Services and Medical/Health Service programs, Washtenaw County Community Mental Health, Ann Arbor, MI.

Edward Marks, PhD, Executive Director of United Behavioral Systems, Georgia, Atlanta, GA.

Robin L. Michaelson, MSc, Public Health Analyst, National Institute of Mental Health Office of Programs for the Homeless Mentally Ill, Rockville, MD.

Bert Pepper, MD, Founder and Executive Director of The Information Exchange (TIE), Inc., New City, NY.

David A. Pollack, MD, Adjunct Associate Professor, Department of Psychiatry, Oregon Health Sciences University, and Medical Director of Mental Health Services West, Portland, OR.

Hilary Ryglewicz, ACSW, Clinical Assistant to the Commissioner of Mental Health and Coordinator of Family/Consumer Services at Rockland County (New York) Department of Mental Health; Training/Publications Coordinator for The Information Exchange (TIE), Inc. and Contributing Editor of its quarterly bulletin *TIE-LINES*, New York City, NY.

James W. Stockdill, PhD, Deputy Director of the Maryland Mental Hygiene Administration, Baltimore, MD.

Table of Contents

Innovations
in
Community
Mental Health

1

A Historical Overview of Community Mental Health Centers in the United States

David L. Cutler

ROOTS OF COMMUNITY MENTAL HEALTH IN AMERICA

In his 1963 address to the 88th Congress, John F. Kennedy proposed

> a national mental health program to assist in the inauguration of a wholly new emphasis and approach to care for the mentally ill. Central to a new mental health program is comprehensive community care. We need a new type of health care facility; one which will return mental health care to the mainstream of American medicine, and at the same time upgrade mental health services. I recommend, therefore, that the Congress: #1, Authorize grants to the states for the construction of comprehensive community mental health centers; #2, Authorize short term project grants for the initial staffing costs of comprehensive mental health centers, and, #3, To facilitate the preparation of community plans for these new facilities as a necessary preliminary to any construction or staffing assistance, appropriate 4.2 million dollars for planning grants under the NIMH. (pp. 3-5)

Indeed this was a "bold new approach." The federal government of the United States had decided for the first time since President Pierce vetoed the "National Mental Health Act" of 1854 that in addition to the states it, too, had a role in the direct delivery of mental health services. It was, in essence, a milestone in the history of society's attempts to deal with mentally ill persons.

Although this event seemed like the beginning, it was really the culmination of a chain of social, political, and economic events that characterized the development of programs for the mentally ill throughout the 19th and 20th centuries in America (Maudlin, 1976b). From the East Cambridge, Massachusetts, jail where Dorothea Dix began her national crusade in the mid-1800s (Maudlin, 1976a) to the mental hygiene movement established in the early 20th century by Clifford Beers (1921) and Adolph Meyer (1915), the history of mental health in America had long since established its institutional to noninstitutional movement as a swinging pendulum.

Unfortunately, in the late 19th to early 20th century, the pendulum swung back toward the institution, and the early hopes and dreams of the moral treatment era and Dorothea Dix failed to materialize for the nation's chronically mentally ill. The mental hygiene movement in the early part of the century had only a small impact that resulted in the development of a few child guidance clinics and psychopathic hospitals. Nonetheless, these ideas had their impact on American psychiatry, particularly the work of Adolph Meyer, Eric Lindemann, and later Gerald Caplan, whose *Principles of Preventive Psychiatry* (1963) formed the basis of the conceptual development of the community mental health movement in America.

THE COMMUNITY
MENTAL HEALTH REVOLUTION

Prior to World War II the federal government played an almost insignificant role in the development and management of mental health programs in the United States. The first major piece of legislation that specifically addressed the problem of the mentally ill in America was the National Mental Health Act (Public Law 79-487) which was passed in July of 1946. This legislation created the National Institute of Mental Health (NIMH) which was to become the think tank and the financial source for much of the innovative mental health programming that was to follow in the next three decades. The Act provided for NIMH to provide technical assistance and consultation to states to enable them to set up a single mental health authority. The Act also established research and training grant programs that continue to exist.

In the 1950s several crucial events occurred whose effects cannot entirely be separated from one another. First, in 1955 there appeared to be a peak in the nation's population of patients in mental hospitals. Following that year the population began to diminish. This decrease was associated temporally with the development of therapeutic communities in the state hospitals (J. Cumming & E. Cumming, 1962; Jones, 1953) and the discovery of major tranquilizers. Also, increasing numbers of mental health practitioners and facilities appeared in the community. From a high of nearly 600,000 in American state hospitals in 1955, the population declined to about 200,000 in 1975. As this process developed, it became more and more apparent that something needed to be done with these long-term mentally ill persons now in the community if they were no longer to live in the hospital. As a result, in 1958 the United States Congress passed the Mental Health Study Act (Public Law 84-192) to provide for "an objective, thorough, and nationwide analysis and reevaluation of the human and economic problems of mental illness" (Joint Commission on Mental Illness and Mental Health, 1961, p. 301).

As a part of the final report of this commission in 1961, a book was published, entitled *Action for Mental Health* (Appel & Bartemeier, 1961). This book described needs for a new sort of mental health system, staffing patterns, costs, and methods. Of course, in 1961 John F. Kennedy had become President, and, having had personal experience with mental disability in his own family, he was not at all unreceptive to these ideas. On February 5th, 1963, President Kennedy spoke to the Congress about mental health and retardation. It was during this speech that he proposed a new National Mental Health Program as well as the appropriation of 4.2 million dollars for planning grants to be distributed by the National Institute of Mental Health. Kennedy thought that this new program could eventually result in the phasing out of state hospitals all over the country and the substitution of high quality treatment in the patient's local community.

There was an emphasis on community involvement and community ownership of the program. In addition, the programs were to be comprehensive, providing services not only to the severely mentally ill, but also to children, families, and adults suffering from the effects of stress. These programs were to be comprehensive, coordinated, of high quality, and available to the total population. In essence, where this country had failed to establish a comprehensive national health service or national health insurance system, the President was now proposing exactly that for mental health systems. As we shall see, these goals remain largely unachieved.

THE KENNEDY-JOHNSON YEARS (1961-1969)

The early years of the community mental health movement were marked by great expectations, much optimism, and rapid development. However, it is important to recognize that very little actually happened during Kennedy's administration. Legislation seemed stuck in Congress for 9 months between February, the time Kennedy gave his address, and October 31, 1963, the date he signed the Community Mental Health Centers Act into law. The original Act contained no provision for staffing the centers, only allocations for buildings. Many powerful lobby groups, including the American Medical Association, were opposed to prepaid or government-paid health plans. In addition, many members of Congress were concerned about the federal government building and staffing these new facilities in local communities and then expecting the local communities to pick up the funding for them 4 years later. As a result, the staffing portion of the bill was deleted, and only the Construction Act was passed in 1963. Less than a month after he signed the Act, President Kennedy was assassinated, and it fell to Lyndon Johnson's administration to develop the funding amendments for staff, which were finally passed in August of 1965. It was generally felt at the time that passing the staffing portion of the Mental Health Act was to a large extent accomplished out of sentiment for John F. Kennedy. However, beginning in 1965 and extending until 1970, federally designated mental health catchment areas (of 100,000 to 200,000 people) all over the country began applying for federal grants.

The first federal grant was awarded to Winter Haven, Florida, Hospital Community Mental Health Center (CMHC) in October of 1965. Altogether 10 grants were funded in 1965, including six in California alone. Many of the first grants were associated with hospitals and were responsible for building new wings on old hospitals. However, the intent of the community mental health legislation was to assure that communities themselves appointed boards and controlled the mental health centers.

Hospital boards came to be suspect as not being truly representative of the community. Consequently, later amendments to the Mental Health Centers Act spelled out more clearly the role and composition of mental health center boards to assure that they truly reflected the ethnic, racial, and demographic profiles of the community.

Many of the amendments to the Act were quite complicated; I will try to simplify them by discussing primarily the requirements for services. The original centers were required to provide inpatient and outpatient services as well as consultation and education, day treatment, and crisis services. The amendments of 1968 provided the addition of alcohol and drug abuse services. In 1970, Congress again modified the Act to include children as needing mental health care. This was a direct response to the report of the Joint Commission on Mental Health of Children (1969). In 1970 the Act was amended to provide for 8 years of funding instead of only 4. The federal portion of the funding was set at 75% for the first 2 years, 60% for the 3rd year, 45% for the 4th year, and 30% for the remaining 4 years. In addition, the government added a new priority of poverty as a main feature for competition for funding. The poverty area centers could get 90% of the costs of construction paid for by federal funds. The federal government would also pay for 90% of staffing costs for the first 2 years, 80% in the 3rd year, 75% in the 4th year, and 70% for the remaining 4 years. This was a significant advantage for poverty centers.

GROWTH AND CONSOLIDATION (1969-1976)

Although the Nixon and Ford administrations were certainly not supportive of mental health legislation and funding, community programs nonetheless thrived during those years due to the presence of a persistent Democratic majority in the Congress. In 1974 Congress offered an additional series of amendments that would increase the comprehensiveness of the service spectrum. Under the provision of this law all new and existing centers were required to provide five services that had been deemed essential from the beginning of the mental health movement (Bloom, 1977). These included inpatient, outpatient, partial hospitalization, emergency services, and consultation and education. Second, services to children and the elderly were required, which were to include diagnostic, treatment, liaison, and follow-up elements. Third, consultation and education services were to continue to community agencies, courts, police, other physicians, public welfare, and so on. Fourth, mental health centers were required to screen for persons being considered for admission to a public psychiatric facility to determine if the admission would be necessary. Fifth, follow-up services such as halfway houses were made mandatory. And sixth, programs for prevention, treatment, and rehabilitation of alcohol or other drug abuse could be required if the federal government considered these services necessary.

Although in 1974 President Ford did veto the extension of the Community Mental Health Act, existing centers were supported by congressional continuing resolutions until a new bill could be developed in 1975. This new extension was also vetoed by President Ford on the grounds that it was too expensive, but this time Congress was able to override the veto by a wide margin and Public Law 94-63 was passed. Once again new programs could be funded on the now 8-year decreasing funds formula. Between 1968 and 1975 a total of 445 CMHCs were funded (60% of all centers funded 1965-1980; Smith, 1984).

This era also marked a change in geographic distribution in patterns of establishing new centers from the East Coast and California to the South and the Great Plains. Nonetheless, despite a significant percentage of catchment areas participating, many states were very reluctant to get involved in the federal initiative at all. They reasoned that once the federal government backed out after the 8 year start-up period they would be left holding the bag for the continuing costs (not such bad reasoning). Consequently, when the program was dropped by the Reagan administration in 1981, only 754 of a possible 1,500 eligible catchment areas nationwide had actually applied for and received funding. Furthermore, in the final phase (1975-1980), actual federal dollars were reduced while inflation more than doubled the cost of construction as well as staffing costs, so that the impact of the remaining funding was considerably less. After 1975 no new construction was attempted due largely to prohibitive costs. Two hundred and eighteen centers were funded during this phase, including several in Oregon, which was one of those states that had been very cautious about taking federal support. Ironically, since the block grant legislation took effect, Oregon has been able to retain its share of federal funding relatively intact for the next 12 years, even after the revolving fund formula of decreasing federal support no longer applied.

PROGRAM PLANNING AND
CONFLICT IN COMMUNITY MENTAL HEALTH

Several principles soon became apparent in the evolution of this new community mental health industry. For one thing, each community mental health center was located in a setting that had its own characteristics and belief systems. Rural programs were quite different from urban programs and also quite different from each other. Every community had a different set of problems that provided the backdrop within which mental illness could be viewed. With deinstitutionalization taking place, inner cities and small towns that happened to have state hospitals tended to collect the chronically mentally ill. Suburban areas where rapid growth was taking place tended to fill up with rootless people who had very little capacity to effectively handle the stress of multiple changing life events. Rural areas where small farms were being bought up and converted into large agribusinesses developed serious transgenerational conflicts where the sons could no longer find opportunities to work the farms as their fathers had before them. In these areas, alcoholism became a major epidemiological problem. Mental health center boards and executive directors were faced with having to plan mental health services for their catchment area, but were given only a limited range of activities that their staffs were authorized to engage in. In addition, many rural clinics had problems with transportation, and many urban ones developed labor-management disputes.

Beyond the difficulty of adapting community mental health clinics to specific settings and patient populations, multiple issues developed from a lack of understanding of the need to plan collaboratively with existing agencies that were already providing services of various sorts to these populations. This included not only the public sector, but also a very large American private sector. Counseling services were not only the domain of psychiatry and psychology, but also clergy, lay therapists, pharmacists, attorneys, nonpsychiatric physicians, and other townsfolk who might be referred to as "natural helpers." Community mental health centers were the "new kids on the block," and as such many of them managed to step on everyone's toes rather than develop working relationships with everyone. Centers were, in fact, set up in direct competition with state hospitals and were labeled as an alternative to the state hospitals. However, most of these centers were staffed by people who were much more interested in insight-oriented psychotherapy with neurotics than in case management or rehabilitation of schizophrenics. Consequently, although chronically mentally ill persons were leaving the hospitals, they were not always picked up for follow-up by the community mental health centers.

Many centers felt that the really important goal was to prevent mental illness in the first place. Ambitious primary prevention projects were developed that were thought to reduce the incidence of mental illness, but they were rarely evaluated to ascertain their effectiveness. Most centers, however, were able to form good crisis intervention services. In some states these took the form of mobile crisis teams in addition to "hot lines" and walk-in clinics. Although the basic services required by the federal government had always included emergency crisis services, these were generally thought of as being crisis intervention for less than mentally ill people, to prevent them from becoming mentally ill. Centers were surprised to find out that most of the people using the crisis and emergency services turned out to be not only already mentally ill, but also significantly disabled as well!

DAY TREATMENT

Because there was a strong bias toward avoiding hospitalization, day hospitals began to develop as major program elements in the mental health centers. The first day hospitals were just that - hospital milieus that were transferred into the community. These were certainly congruent with the original CMHC federal guidelines of "partial hospitalization." These programs were essentially therapeutic community-oriented programs staffed by traditional hospital personnel and set up for the sole purpose of avoiding hospitalization for those patients who did not require a bed in the hospital overnight. Patients were guided from group to group from 9:00 in the morning to 3:30 in the afternoon on a 5-day-a-week basis. Programs tended to consist of talk groups, with some rest periods in between.

A nice example of this sort of day program was one that existed in the Southern Arizona Mental Health Center from 1970 to 1985 (Beigel, 1972). In this program patients were hospitalized at the local county hospital, the psychiatrist-director of the mental health center went to the hospital, staffed all the patients between 6:00 a.m. and 8:00 a.m., and those patients who were able to leave the hospital for milieu therapy programs were placed on a bus and sent to the mental health center several miles away. When the patients were ready to leave the hospital they were already well connected to a mental health center and continued to attend day treatment for the next 2 or 3 months until they were stabilized enough to be managed in general outpatient care. This form of "hospital" day treatment provided an excellent supportive environment in which patients could slowly reconstitute, especially those who already had a reasonable place to live and did not require 24-hour supervision. It was extremely effective in reducing utilization of hospital beds, and may have been the single most cost-effective form of day treatment developed during the community mental health movement.

However, several other types of day treatment became necessary and considerably more in vogue in the mid- to late 1970s. Each had a somewhat different focus, model, and effect. Whereas the day hospital was, in fact, a substitute for hospital, later day programs took on more of a rehabilitation focus. For example, the adult development program in Seattle, Washington, was set up entirely as a college for mentally ill persons. Patients enrolled as students and took classes in such things as precision behavior change, mood modification, emotional growth through drama, dance therapy, and so on. These patients received a diploma when they graduated and were eventually asked to join an alumni group. Patients were even given the opportunity to major in a particular mental health subject. Their case workers were not called therapists, but instead were called counselors. This particular model became very popular in the late 1970s and spread to many parts of the country. It was quite useful for relatively stable persons, some of whom were chronically mentally ill, but most of whom had personality disorders and mild affective disorders.

Some patients were not seen as being capable of responding to educational models - growth-oriented day treatment programs. For these patients it was felt that a program should be designed that was purely sustenance and support oriented. An example of these was the Community Organization for Personal Enrichment program developed in Tucson - a system of church-based socialization centers where patients went primarily for fellowship. Here volunteers from local churches mingled with patients who were involved in aftercare in the local mental health clinics. Consultation was provided on a weekly basis by center staff to the volunteers who then dealt with the patients (Cutler & Beigel, 1978). A similar program was developed in Massachusetts, where the state provided funding for social clubs that were operated by the patients themselves. The goal of these programs was merely social support, not growth. The patients were accepted under practically any condition as long as they were not violent. These programs were very important as an adjunct to the state hospitals, because all patients needed somewhere to go and somewhere to belong following their discharge from the hospital (Cutler, 1979; Cutler, Tatum, & Shore, 1987).

A fourth and perhaps the most sophisticated form of day program was the earliest form of the psychosocial rehabilitation model. This was primarily patterned after the Fountain House program in New York, which had been in existence since the 1940s (Beard, 1979). Here members start out in the social club environment and work their way up to temporary employment positions. In these situations they share jobs with other members and are able to gain tremendous self-esteem knowing that they are able to contribute by doing a job for which they get paid. This particular model of day treatment is now considered mainstream, and most day treatment programs throughout the country use some form of this within their basic model.

CLINICAL ISSUES IN COMMUNITY MENTAL HEALTH

Although at the time it was thought that a great deal of skill existed among the various professional disciplines to provide services for mentally ill persons in community mental health centers, it is clear now that those skills did not exist and did not develop until quite recently. Consequently, during the 1960s and 1970s, community mental health centers opened, hired large numbers of professional staff, and began doing things that, although well intentioned, often were irrelevant to the needs of the patient population that they were dealing with. It is safe to say that very few mental health centers evaluated their work, so that for the most part they managed to remain unaware of the ineffectiveness of what they were doing. Most community mental health center staff called themselves psychotherapists. However, few of them had had intensive training in their academic environments in psychotherapy. Many learned their skills through workshops and training events that occurred following the achievement of their degrees. However, what they learned was primarily adaptable to relatively high-functioning neurotic people and not to the ever-increasing numbers of young chronically mentally ill persons who were in need of services. People became skilled as family therapists, but few thought of themselves as social skills trainers, case managers, prevocational trainers, home visitors, and so forth. Consequently, until the mid-1970s the major target populations served by most mental health centers were children, families, depressed persons, and so on. Chronically mentally ill people were seen in the mental health centers, but were seen primarily by the psychiatrists, who often only saw them for 15 minutes and wrote prescriptions. Some centers hired general practitioners and nurse practitioners who saw people at an even more rapid pace. The physicians on the whole did a good job, but generally speaking did not get a great deal of help with this group from the others. Chronically mentally ill people continued to be ill but no longer had hospitals and their staffs to look after them.

THE REEMERGENCE OF THE
CHRONIC MENTAL PATIENT

Despite the rapid growth of community mental health centers throughout the country, the plight of the chronic mental patient continued to be relatively neglected. Mental health centers, smitten with grandiose ideas of preventing mental health problems before they started, developed prevention programs, crisis clinics, and psychotherapy clinics for the masses. In their haste to create comprehensive care for entire communities they somehow forgot to think about long-term care for the chronic patient. During the heyday of rapid growth of community mental health centers in the 1960s and 1970s the chronic patients continued to get their care either in state hospitals or in state hospital aftercare clinics, which for the most part remained totally separate from community mental health centers. In fact, with few exceptions, mental health centers and state hospitals operated as totally independent administrative entities, deriving their funding from entirely different sources. State hospitals were dependent on state legislators for funding; community mental health centers received their staffing grants from the federal government and were able to capture a variety of local funds including third-party payments. It was as if there were two systems. As deinstitutionalization progressed it became apparent that this situation could not continue to exist.

11

RESEARCH AND
EVALUATION OF MODEL PROGRAMS

A few model programs that advocated cooperation and collaboration between hospitals and CMHCs had begun to develop in the late 1960s. These included the Fort Logan Mental Health Center in Denver, Colorado (Pollack & Kirby, 1976); Southern Arizona Mental Health Center in Tucson, Arizona (Beigel, 1972); the Program for Assertive Community Treatment (PACT) in Madison, Wisconsin (Stein, Test, & Marx, 1975); and the Living in the Community program in Pendleton, Oregon (Cutler et al., 1984). These programs, along with several others (Bachrach, 1980) were successful in dealing with the chronically mentally ill because they redeployed state hospital resources for community programs. As long as the staff of these programs were successful in maintaining chronic patients in reasonably decent living situations in the community neither the patients nor the staff had to go back to the state hospital (Cutler, 1983).

Perhaps the best known of these programs was the PACT program in Madison, Wisconsin (Stein & Test, 1976), which actually deinstitutionalized an entire ward, including staff, by moving them into the community with their patients. They were assigned basically the same tasks in the community that they had done in the hospital. The program was considered highly successful in helping patients adapt to the community and spawned the best known research done in community mental health (Stein & Test, 1980).

THE COMMUNITY SUPPORT PROGRAM

As a result of the success of these model programs, NIMH became interested in finding some method of reproducing them throughout the country. NIMH began in the early 1970s by examining the problems facing the deinstitutionalized chronic mental patient, but it was not until 1977 that 19 states and the District of Columbia began receiving NIMH contracts for a new "Community Support Program" (CSP) designed to implant a framework within state mental health planning authorities that would specifically target the system toward the chronic mental patient. Funds became available to study these various model programs or other demonstration projects, so as to disseminate information gleaned from these projects (Turner & Shifren,

1979). In addition, funds were also made available to state agencies for planning projects that would assess the needs of the CSP population; identify the ways in which CSP components could be provided; clarify who was responsible for providing such services; and take the steps necessary to fill gaps, improve coordination, and upgrade quality.

There were initially 19 grants in 1977, and by 1982 almost all the states received some sort of community support planning grant from the federal government. The intent of these grants was to get the state, the federal government, and local programs working collaboratively to provide services to this high priority group of patients. In the late 1970s, NIMH regional offices, working collaboratively with the training and manpower branch at the central office, began funding specialized training at schools of social work, nursing, psychiatry, and psychology for work with chronic patients (Cutler, Bloom, & Shore, 1981).

Methodology for case management, social skills training, network building, and resource development were taught to existing CMHC staff at NIMH-sponsored learning communities throughout the country. Funds were also provided to pay expenses for staff to travel to model programs and observe their methods. These included the Fountain House Psychosocial Rehabilitation Club in New York, PACT in Wisconsin, and South West Denver Community Mental Health Center. Although these projects were not designed as research, they were extremely effective in disseminating methodology and ideology to other states and within states to shape the public system to the needs of the chronically mentally ill and also to some degree to the exclusion of the not-so-chronically mentally ill (Cutler et al., 1984).

THE PRESIDENT'S COMMISSION ON MENTAL HEALTH

Concerned with the fate of chronic mental patients, and having successfully presided over the development of an advanced program in Georgia, President Carter in 1976 appointed his wife, Rosalyn, to head the President's Commission on Mental Health. This commission traveled to various places throughout the country examining the plight of a variety of target populations of mentally ill persons including the chronically mentally ill. The commission held public hearings in four states in 1977. In addition, task force members visited hundreds of facilities throughout the country and solicited responses from professionals and from thousands of citizens whose lives had been affected by persons with mental or emotional disabilities.

The report found, in essence, that despite a massive increase in community services over the previous 15 years, many groups continued to be largely unserved or underserved. These included racial and ethnic minorities, the urban poor, migrant and seasonal farm workers, women, Vietnam veterans, the deaf and others with physical handicaps, and, of course, children, adolescents, and adults with chronic mental illness. They found only a few communities that had a broad range of community-based services including halfway houses, foster and group homes, and community mental health centers. For the most part, however, they heard an enormous amount of testimony and reports regarding persons with chronic mental disabilities who had been released from the hospital but who simply lacked the basic necessities of life. These people had no adequate housing, no adequate clothing, and no adequate food. Follow-up mental health aftercare and general medical care were woefully lacking. In addition, half of the people released from large mental hospitals were being readmitted within a year of discharge. This report was highly discouraging, considering the amount of time, money, and effort that had been spent on developing community mental health centers.

The report recommended dramatic efforts to increase the strength of natural support networks in the community and link those support networks to formal mental health services. They recommended that a national priority be established to meet the needs of people with chronic mental illness and that services be developed in close collaboration with other health and human service agencies. The report also recommended the development of a new federal grant program for community mental health services that would give priority to underserved and unserved populations, particularly children, adolescents, the elderly, and racial and ethnic minorities. It recommended appropriating at least 75 million dollars in the first year and 100 million dollars in each of the next 2 years. In addition, it recommended the development of a national plan to serve as a frame of reference for developing programs for the mentally ill.

Most of these recommendations were incorporated into the new National Mental Health Systems Act (1980). The main features of this new Act were (a) priority given to vulnerable groups such as the chronically mentally ill, children, adolescents, and the elderly; (b) a restructuring of federal, state, and local relationships allowing the states more control of the management and distribution of federal funds coming to local programs; (c) an emphasis on planning, including performance contracts with each program as a condition of federal funding; (d) enhancement of linkages between mental health and general health care facilities focusing on the prevention of mental illness; and (e) an increase in advocacy services for the mentally ill.

Altogether approximately 800 million new dollars were authorized in addition to the continuation costs for the already funded and existing community mental health centers. The Mental Health Systems Act was a more conservative version of the 1963 Mental Health Centers Construction Act; it was designed in some degree to restructure the system and focus it more on underserved and severely ill populations as well as to include the states more meaningfully in decision making about who received funds.

THE NEW AMERICAN FEDERALISM

Unfortunately, in January, 1981, President Reagan chose to have nothing to do with this new law. He recommended a cut of 25% off the top of all CMHC funding immediately, and then to convert all the federal funds into block grant monies to be distributed to the states to do with pretty much as they would like (Buck, 1984). In fact, in August of 1981, President Reagan signed into law the Omnibus Budget Reconciliation Act that essentially eliminated all of the carefully developed federal initiatives of the previous 18 years in one huge budget-cutting action. Although 75% of the original community mental health centers' money was left intact, all of the additional Mental Health Systems Act money was written off, and in the ensuing months enormous cuts in NIMH central and regional offices resulted in a complete lack of capacity on the part of the federal government to process, supervise, site visit, and provide technical assistance to already existing federal community mental health centers throughout the country.

By 1982, all of the 10 federal regional offices of NIMH were closed, cutting out 400 positions, and support for services dropped from 293 million dollars in 1980 to 203 million dollars in 1982 (Foley & Sharfstein, 1983). As Estes and Wood pointed out (1984), many mental health centers have had to counteract the loss of federal funding by increasing their fees and reducing staffing and services. They reported that 31% of all CMHCs that they contacted had indicated that their service capacity was reduced

15

due to staffing losses. In addition to this, there were longer waiting lists and decreased quality of services.

Thompson and Bass (1984) also pointed out that there were
rather dramatic changes in CMHC staffing patterns. In particular, their study found a decrease in numbers of psychiatrists,
nurses, and other clinical staff. There was an increase in the
number of master's level psychologists and social workers. This
is, of course, consistent with a great deal of earlier literature that
describes the demedicalization of community mental health centers.

Citing data compiled by the National Institute of Mental
Health for the period of 1970-1975, Winslow (1979) concluded
that psychiatrists were leaving CMHCs and were being replaced
by other mental health professionals. Langsley and Robinowitz
(1979) described the growing antimedical attitudes in community
mental health centers and the inclination of psychiatrists to work
in settings similar to their original training sites as being barriers
to psychiatric involvement in community mental health centers.
Talbott (1979) observed that the flight of psychiatrists from the
public sector coincided with increased public funding of private
and voluntary not-for-profit facilities through Medicare, Medicaid, and other means. Beigel (1984), on the other hand, describes
strategies to remedicalize community mental health centers given
the tremendous need of the chronically mentally ill to have psychiatric evaluation and treatment. He postulated that forensic
issues, psychopharmacologic issues, and medical issues would
drive centers toward recruiting more psychiatrists in the future.

How has community mental health coped with this major
regressive series of events? Generally, a number of things have
happened. For one thing, the centers have become more focused
on the chronically mentally ill. No longer do they have the luxury
of treating the broad spectrum of psychological problems, neurotic disorders, crises, and the like. They are now forced to treat
only the severely mentally ill. In addition they have had to reduce
staffing patterns, increase clinical case loads, cut back overall levels of services, and, in essence, centralize their operations. There
is also a greater reliance on fees than there has been in the past.
Centers are particularly interested in recouping Medicare and
Medicaid payments as well as competing with the private sector
for the business of persons who have insurance policies. Centers
are also becoming more extensively used as training sites for a
variety of mental health professional disciplines. This could also
be a reflection of the cuts in funds for training, forcing psychiatry,

nursing psychology, and social work programs to turn to community mental health centers for support (Faulkner et al., 1982; Okin, 1984).

Unfortunately, despite the refocus of state resources on the chronic and severely mentally ill, rising costs and rising numbers of "baby boomers" reaching adulthood have overwhelmed both state hospitals and CMHCs. Bigelow et al. (1988) point out that state hospitals are filling up and backing up with hard to place patients who are too much for CMHCs to deal with despite their best efforts. Not only are hospitals overfilled, there is now also an enormous problem with homeless mentally ill in the United States (Lamb, 1984).

FUNDING MENTAL HEALTH CARE IN AMERICA IN THE 1990s

One of the most difficult aspects of understanding the array of services available in the United States is the peculiar maze of entitlement programs and eligibility requirements. The majority of Americans are served by private insurance programs generally paid for by the companies they work for. A few of the affluent who do not work are able to pay their own insurance premiums. People with less severe mental problems who can work generally have reasonable coverage for health, but mental health coverage is almost always limited in some way. For example, currently in the state of Oregon insurance companies do not have to provide more than $7,500 in coverage for inpatient care and no more than $2,000 for outpatient care in a 2-year period. At 1990 rates this would cover no more than 15 days in a biennium for inpatient and about 20 hours of outpatient psychotherapy.

Veterans who were injured in service are eligible for free services for life as long as they are considered service connected. In addition, they may also receive large pensions depending upon how disabled they are in social and vocational functioning. Although other nondisabled veterans may also receive services, they are low priority and may receive care only on a space-available basis, if at all. Currently, the Veterans' Administration is cutting back on services, thereby driving more nonservice-connected vets into CMHCs.

Since the advent of federal Medicaid (health payments for the poor) and Medicare (payment for care of the elderly) the large public hospitals that previously existed in most cities and counties have been sold off by local governments; many are now private facilities. In order to remain financially solvent they must now collect third-party payments from insurance companies, Medicare and Medicaid, and state and local welfare. Since these payments do not cover the entire cost of care, they either have to raise their rates to private patients or avoid serving the poor. Although most poor people are eligible for public welfare, if they have substantial savings or an income of more than $300 to $400 per month, they will be denied any health or mental health coverage whatsoever. The result of this confusing and complicated privatization of the public system is that some people either have to lie to obtain eligibility or be a part of an estimated 40 million people who have no health coverage at all (Paulson, 1988). Many of these people are turned away when they come for help even in emergencies.

Gerald Caplan (R. Caplan & G. Caplan, 1969) has said:

> In a democratic capitalist country, individual psychiatrists have the freedom to decide how they will use their skills and make a living, but as corporate professionals they must either be responsive to organized communal demands to deal with formally recognized population needs or they will incur sanctions and eventually be pushed aside in favor of some other profession, the development of which will be fostered in order to deal with the neglected problem. (p. 320)

G. Caplan also pointed out that "community psychiatrists who are not competent physicians are not likely to make optimal and effective contributions to community mental health planning" (p. 346). Clinical skills and administrative skills go together and cannot be divorced from one another.

G. Caplan's first statement has certainly come true to a large extent in the United States; that is, psychiatry as a profession no longer occupies a leadership position with respect to assuring that the mental health needs of the masses are met. Although other professions have risen to fill the void left by a lack of administratively skilled psychiatrists, they too have overlooked the need for clinical expertise to be a part of the planning process. Clinical issues, quality of care, and so on, get lost in the shuffle as business oriented administrators are hired to replace social workers and psychologists to turn these clinics into profit-making operations. John Talbott, president of the American Psychiatric Association between 1984 and 1985, said in 1985:

I believe strongly that the future of the public system of
care and treatment of the severely and chronically mentally ill will be ensured only if we take as our primary
focus the recipients of all of our treatment activity and
energies -- our patients. We cannot allow government's
fixation on bricks and mortar, or third party reimburse-
ments obsession with cost-cutting to override what is right
for the mentally ill. (p. 50)

Talbott's leadership in the quest for clinically sound and accessible programs for the chronically mentally ill has been encouraging given the demoralizing period we are in. We hope that the
1990s will bring a rebirth of energy into the public sector effort.
Unfortunately, we may be faced with more unrealistic solutions.

In a tongue-in-cheek article published in the bicentennial
(July 1976) issue of the journal of *Hospital and Community Psychiatry*, Eugene Resnick (1976) wrote about mental health in the
future. His chilling description of his visit to Madame Futura and
her predictions are not only classic but seem to be coming true!

In 1988, she told me as she peered into her cathode tube,
mental illness was all but conquered in the U.S.A. It had
been done very simply - by appropriate legislation. President Donald Degan and Congress, now dominated by the
Patriotic American Party, decided that mental illness was
a luxury the country no longer could afford. Tax money
was required for essential services, such as national defense against foreign ideologies, so all appropriations for
psychiatric facilities, training, and research were eliminated. It was quite clear that with the closing of all clinics
and the anticipated (by 1998) closing of all state psychiatric hospitals, mental illness too would be eliminated. (p.
520)

David L. Cutler, MD, is Professor of Psychiatry and Director of
the Public Psychiatry Training Program, Department of Psychiatry, Oregon Health Sciences University in Portland, Oregon. He is also the editor of the *Community Mental Health
Journal.* Dr. Cutler can be contacted at Department of Psychiatry, Oregon Health Sciences University, 3181 Sam Jackson
Park Road, Portland, OR 97201.

REFERENCES

Appel, K. E., & Bartemeier, L. H. (1961). *Action for Mental Health: Final Report of the Joint Commission on Mental Illness and Health.* New York: Basic Books.

Bachrach, L. L. (1980). Overview: Model programs for chronic mental patients. *American Journal of Psychiatry, 137,* 1023-1031.

Beard, J. H. (1979). The rehabilitation services of Fountain House. In L. I. Stein & M. A. Test (Eds.), *Alternatives to Mental Hospital Treatment* (pp. 201-215). New York: Plenum Press.

Beers, C. (1921). *A Mind That Found Itself.* New York: Doubleday.

Beigel, A. (1972, August). Alternatives to psychiatric hospitalization: The Pima County combined mental health care program experience. *Arizona Medicine, 29,* 642-645.

Beigel, A. (1984). The remedicalization of community mental health. *Hospital and Community Psychiatry, 35,* 1114-1117.

Bigelow, D. A., Cutler, D. L., Moore, L. J., McComb, P., & Leung, P. (1988). Characteristics of state hospital patients who are hard to place. *Hospital and Community Psychiatry, 39,* 181-185.

Bloom, B. L. (1977). *Community Mental Health, a General Introduction.* Monterey, CA: Brooks/Cole.

Buck, J. A. (1984). Block grants and federal promotion of community mental health services, 1946-1964. *Community Mental Health Journal, 20,* 236-247.

Caplan, G. (1963). *Principles of Preventive Psychiatry.* New York: Basic Books.

Caplan, R., & Caplan, G. (1969). *History of Psychiatry in the 19th Century.* New York: Basic Books.

Cumming, J., & Cumming, E. (1962). *Ego and Milieu.* New York: Atherton Press.

Cutler, D. L. (1979). Volunteer support networks for chronic patients. In L. I. Stein (Ed.), *Community Support Systems for the Long Term Patient* (pp. 67-74). San Francisco: Jossey-Bass.

Cutler, D. L. (1983). The Pima County approach: You call this a system? In Unified Health Systems Unrepaired. In J. Talbott (Ed.), *New Directions for Mental Health Services* (No. 18, pp. 85-88). San Francisco: Jossey-Bass.

Cutler, D. L., & Beigel, A. (1978). A church-based program of community activities for chronic patients. *Hospital and Community Psychiatry, 29,* 497-501.

Cutler, D. L., Bloom, J. D., & Shore, J. H. (1981). Training psychiatrists to work with community support systems for chronically mentally ill persons. *American Journal of Psychiatry, 138,* 98-101.

Cutler, D. L., Tatum, E., & Shore, J. H. (1987). A comparison of schizophrenic patients in different community support treatment approaches. *Community Mental Health Journal, 23,* 103-113.

Cutler, L. D., Terwilliger, W., Faulkner, L., Field, G., & Bray, D. (1984). Disseminating the principles of a community support program. *Hospital and Community Psychiatry, 35,* 51-55.

Estes, C., & Wood, J. (1984). A preliminary assessment of the impact of block grants on community mental health centers. *Hospital and Community Psychiatry, 35,* 1125-1129.

Faulkner, L. R., Eaton, J. S., Bloom, J. D., & Cutler, D. L. (1982). The CMHC as a setting for residency education. *Community Mental Health Journal, 18,* 3-10.

Foley, H. A., & Sharfstein, S. S. (1983). *Madness in Government: Who Cares for the Mentally Ill?* Washington, DC: American Psychiatric Press.

Jones, M. (1953). *The Therapeutic Community.* New York: Basic Books.

Kennedy, J. F. (1963). *Message from the President of the United States Relative to Mental Illness and Mental Retardation* (88th Cong., 1st Ses., Doc. 58). Washington, DC: U.S. Government Printing Office.

Lamb, H. R. (1984). *The Homeless Mentally Ill* (A task force report). Washington, DC: American Psychiatric Association.

Langsley, D. G., & Robinowitz, C. B. (1979). Psychiatric manpower: An overview. *Hospital and Community Psychiatry, 30,* 749-755.

Maudlin, H. (1976a). Dorothea Lynde Dix, crusader on behalf of the mentally ill. *Hospital and Community Psychiatry, 27,* 471-472.

Maudlin, H. (1976b). Moral treatment in America's lunatic asylums. *Hospital and Community Psychiatry, 277,* 468-470.

Meyer, A. (1915). Objective psychology or psychobiology with subordination of the medically useless contrast of mental and physical. *Journal of the American Medical Association, 65,* 860-862.

21

Okin, R. L. (1984). How community mental health centers are coping. *Hospital and Community Psychiatry, 35,* 1118-1125.

Paulson, R. I. (1988). People and garbage are not the same: Issues in contracting for public mental health services. *Community Mental Health Journal, 25,* 91-102.

Pollack, P., & Kirby, M. (1976). A model to replace psychiatric hospitals. *Journal of Nervous and Mental Disease, 161,* 13-22.

Resnick, E. V. (1976). Mental health care in America (1976). *Hospital and Community Psychiatry, 27,* 519-521.

Smith, C. J. (1984). Geographic patterns of funding for community mental health centers. *Hospital and Community Psychiatry, 35,* 1133-1141.

Stein, L. I., & Test, M. A. (1976). Retaining hospital staff for work in a community program in Wisconsin. *Hospital and Community Psychiatry, 27,* 266-268.

Stein, L. I., & Test, M. A. (1980). Alternatives to mental hospital treatment: Conceptual model, treatment program, and clinical evaluation. *Archives of General Psychiatry, 37,* 392-400.

Stein, L. I., Test, M. A., & Marx, A. J. (1975). Alternatives to mental hospital treatment. Alternative to the hospital: A controlled study. *American Journal of Psychiatry, 132,* 517-522.

Talbott, J. (1979). Why psychiatrists leave the public sector. *Hospital and Community Psychiatry, 3,* 778-782.

Talbott, J. (1985). The fate of the public psychiatry system. *Hospital and Community Psychiatry, 35,* 46-50.

Thompson, J. W., & Bass, R. D. (1984). Changing staffing patterns in community mental health centers. *Hospital and Community Psychiatry, 35,* 1107-1114.

Turner, J. E., & Shifren, L. (1979). Community support systems: How comprehensive? In L. I. Stein (Ed.), *Community Support Systems for the Long Term Patient* (pp. 1-14). San Francisco: Jossey-Bass.

Winslow, W. W. (1979). The changing role of psychiatrists in community mental health centers. *American Journal of Psychiatry, 136,* 24-27.

2

Managed Mental Health Care

Anthony Broskowski
and Edward Marks

Mental health, as a segment of the health care industry, has become the focus of attention over the past few years. While hospital admissions and lengths of stay for medical conditions have declined, utilization of alcohol, drug, and mental health (ADM) care has increased to the point where it now represents 15% to 20% of the medical costs for employers (Wallace, 1987). Although ADM providers have sought to expand their share of the market and revenue base, the employers and insurers who pay for care are seeking to control and manage the escalating costs of ADM services through a variety of cost containment mechanisms (Bagby & Sullivan, 1986).

In this chapter we review the mechanisms being used by various types of managed care systems currently in operation. We then discuss the ways that mental health centers can participate in managed care, paying particular attention to the range and quality of their clinical services and their fiscal and managerial capabilities.

HEALTH CARE COST CONTAINMENT

As they have traditionally done when faced with business-related problems, employers have chosen to begin *managing* all health care costs. Realizing that total health care costs are determined by the formula

Total Costs = Utilization X Cost Per Unit

payors have instituted a range of cost containment mechanisms designed to reduce either the overall rates of utilization or the average price per unit of service (Herzlinger & Calkins, 1986).

When organized in a coherent fashion, these mechanisms constitute various types of "managed care" programs. The primary mechanisms being used to reduce utilization include (a) pretreatment authorization, (b) concurrent utilization review, (c) incentives to receive care from efficient providers, and (d) insurance benefit plans requiring greater employee/user cost sharing. The primary mechanisms used to control price include (a) capitated or negotiated discounted payments to providers, (b) claims review, and (c) insurance coverage for less expensive but equally effective treatment alternatives (Foster-Higgins, 1989).

QUALITY AND COST CONSIDERATIONS

The motivations for managed care systems are not based exclusively on economic factors. Most employers are concerned with the quality of care and are also aware that most persons cannot assess the quality of the care they seek. Furthermore, analysts understand that *cost* and *quality* are related in several ways (Mechanic, 1985; Steffen, 1988). Poor quality care usually leads to additional care, and cost, for the same problems. Fragmented care is often of lower quality, because the synergistic effects of a coordinated system of care are not present.

By managing care, employers hope to enhance clinical effectiveness by encouraging more coordinated, appropriate care. This makes possible a shift in utilization patterns to less restrictive settings, and limits the number of units consumed. Employers are finding that their health and ADM costs can be controlled and in some cases reduced below their currently high levels (Alt, 1988; Fine, 1988).

MECHANISMS USED
IN MANAGED CARE SYSTEMS

Managed care has taken on a number of meanings. To some it means peer review to limit utilization, while others interpret it to require active case management to coordinate and assure continuity of care. In fact, these are only two of the many mechanisms used in managed care systems. We will begin with utilization review mechanisms (Milstein, Oehm, & Alpert, 1987).

PREAUTHORIZATION OF TREATMENT

Preauthorization requires that a provider call a review organization before giving the patient treatment. This initial service review is intended to authorize payment only for that treatment which has been deemed to be "medically necessary and appropriate" (Feldstein, Wickizer, & Wheeler, 1988). Such a mechanism provides a strong incentive for providers to limit care to that which is agreed upon with the external clinical reviewer or gatekeeper.

In most such programs the type and quantity of care that is authorized is based more or less rigidly on some normative value for a particular diagnosis or procedure. Frequently in systems involving mental health and substance abuse, there is considerable discretionary authority given to a professional reviewer to handle each patient episode on a case-by-case basis. Most preauthorization systems give the provider the assurance that if services are authorized they will be paid for, without further review, upon the submission of a valid claim. A provider is not necessarily limited to providing *only* authorized services, although they may risk not being paid for these services and having to bill the patient for some or all of the "unauthorized" care.

Many preauthorization programs assume that the patient will seek services from a provider who will then call the review organization, justify the treatment, and receive the necessary authorizations. However, others offer the employees direct assistance in assessing their medical needs and seeking the "best" provider. Mental health and substance abuse providers will recognize this basic mechanism as an Employee Assistance Program (EAP). In fact, we are now seeing a blending of EAP programs and other types of managed care programs (Bridwell, Collins, & Levine, 1988).

Providers may be concerned that preauthorization control mechanisms could cause reviewers to make decisions based more upon financial constraints than clinical necessity (Melnick & Lyter, 1987). Although abuses can occur, review programs take steps to avoid these conflicts. Reviewers must accept efficient, quality patient care as their highest priority. In addition, procedures usually exist for providers or patients to challenge a reviewer's decisions. If differences of opinion continue to exist, the patient or provider is usually given the opportunity for a third-level review by which the patient, provider, and review program are bound by the decision of an impartial third party (National

Association of Private Psychiatric Hospitals, 1988). The availability of appeals makes it unlikely that financial concerns will take precedence over clinical issues in all of the review mechanisms described in this section.

CONCURRENT UTILIZATION REVIEW

Having sought and received authorization for treatment, how does the employer/insurer/payor know that it is appropriate for the patient to continue in treatment beyond the initial levels of authorized care? In the past, providers were on their own to decide if continued care was necessary. Employers and their insurers have begun extending their review programs to include an *ongoing* review of care, especially for disorders requiring multiple interventions and long-term treatment. Now the fundamental question of ongoing "medical necessity and appropriateness" is being asked of service providers in all settings.

The application of this mechanism generally involves periodic phone calls between a provider and a reviewer, or on-site chart review by a reviewer. The reviewer is seeking continued progress reports and justifications for further extensions in the authorization of services. The reviewer may also assist the provider in a consultative fashion regarding treatment decisions and discharge plans.

As in "preauthorization" programs, the provider is free to continue providing "unauthorized" services, such as maintaining the patient in a hospital when a reviewer has deemed it as no longer "medically necessary or appropriate." The provider remains at all times responsible for the patient's treatment and must make the final decision regarding treatment. They are, however, taking some financial risk to have their claim for payment of unauthorized services denied.

RETROSPECTIVE REVIEW

This mechanism involves the review of a patient's chart by one or more qualified reviewers after the patient is discharged from treatment and a claim for payment has been submitted. The mechanism is only as good as the record keeping involved and does not lend itself to an interactive influence on the quality of care. Such mechanisms, however, continue to be used in conjunction with other types of review, especially when fraud or abuse is suspected.

26

CASE MANAGEMENT

To influence the patient's overall treatment episode, employers and insurers have begun "total case management" mechanisms. Such systems are characterized by a more active and influential professional case manager working collaboratively with one or more providers, spanning multiple treatments, facilities, and time periods.

The use of case management represents a shift in orientation from passive to active involvement. Rather than the provider system responding passively to the requests of the patient, or the review system responding passively to the requests of the provider, the case management system is actively involved in responding to, and on behalf of, the patient and provider. This collaboration leads to greater efficiencies because unnecessary services can be avoided, and the patients receive the level of care best suited to their needs at any given point in time (Brightbill, 1988).

When applied to ADM disorders, case managers may work with the providers, patients, or their families to make sure that the patient receives a comprehensive biopsychosocial assessment resulting in a written treatment plan. Then, based on their authority to approve services and payment, and in some cases to negotiate price or to "flex the benefit" to include services not formally covered in the insurance benefit plan, the case manager undertakes to "triage" the patient to the full range of needed services. Case managers naturally are involved in concurrent review, and collaborate with the providers in determining when one or more services are no longer necessary or appropriate.

*A COMPREHENSIVE NETWORK
OF PROVIDERS AND SERVICES*

If assessment, triage, preauthorization, concurrent review, and case management are to be effective, a comprehensive network of providers and services must be available to address the full range of psychiatric, psychosocial, vocational, and residential needs of a wide variety of potential patients. Ideally, these services will be geographically accessible and available in the evenings or on weekends as well as the usual daytime hours.

The hallmark of a comprehensive psychiatric and substance abuse network will be the availability of *alternatives to 24-hour hospitalization or residential treatment*. Examples of inpatient alternative programs include day and evening outpatient programs for treatment of substance abuse, and day-hospitalization programs for major psychiatric disorders when patient or public safety are not at risk. In-home crisis intervention, with or without therapeutic foster homes, can serve as alternatives to hospitalization for many children and adolescents. There is evidence to suggest that these alternatives are less costly, and that they may be the most effective settings for the patient (Goldstein & Horgan, 1988; Kiesler, 1982; Kiesler & Sibulkin, 1987; Miller & Hester, 1986). By allowing treatment without disrupting other aspects of the patient's life, these alternatives may, in fact, add therapeutic value and facilitate long-term effectiveness.

ALLOCATION OF THE
FINANCIAL RISK FOR TREATMENT

A key mechanism used by most managed care systems is the way they allocate or distribute the financial risks for the cost of providing care among (a) the employee, (b) the patient or user, (c) the provider, (d) the employer, and (e) the managed care organization. The most common methods of allocating costs and risks are as follows:

1. Insurance premiums may be paid for in part by employees, putting part of the cost burden on them whether or not they use medical services.
2. Copayments and deductibles further allocate costs and risks to those who actually use services. Generally there is some maximum limit placed on the user's financial responsibility.
3. The provider assumes risks or contributes to the total cost of care by either (a) agreeing to provide services for a discounted fee or (b) contracting to provide care for a prepaid, per-capita rate.
4. The managed care company, which may be an insurance company or some hybrid utilization review/case management firm, may assume risks by indemnifying the employer for all or some of the cost of care. When assuming all the financial risks, it will retain any savings as profits. The fees paid to the managed care company may be tied to the level of savings achieved, or it may assume responsibility for a percentage of the treatment costs that exceeded an agreed-upon target level. In these cases, it assumes partial risk for the cost of care.

28

5. Historically the employer or insurance company has assumed all or most of the risks of utilization and price. Today most large employers are "self-insured," and directly liable for most of the cost of all insured care, while their "insurance" company is acting in an "administrative services only" (ASO) mode, producing benefit information for employees and doing claims processing for a fee.

CLAIMS REVIEW

Finally, another mechanism that may be present in some managed care systems is the presence of a claims review system. Unlike the traditional "clerical review" of a claim, limited to a determination of an eligible beneficiary receiving an insured service from an eligible provider, claims review in a managed system will also look at the detailed charges and determine if the billed charges match the "authorized services," and at the agreed-upon rates. Claims review will also look for patterns of fraud or abuse, such as services being rendered by an unlicensed provider that are represented as services provided by a licensed colleague.

TYPES OF MANAGED CARE SYSTEMS

In the preceding section we described the specific mechanisms used by managed care systems. In this section, we will describe the major types of managed care systems that currently exist, emphasizing the ways these mechanisms are incorporated or combined.

UTILIZATION REVIEW ORGANIZATIONS (UROs)

Although utilization review was previously discussed as a feature of a managed care system, when offered alone it represents the most rudimentary form of managed care. Utilization review programs are already being used by most major insurers to contain the costs of their entire line of health care coverage. In addition, specialty utilization review firms have now evolved. These firms subcontract to insurers or other managed care systems to apply their review procedures to specified types of care, such as mental health and substance abuse. The most common types of review done by these companies are preadmission certification and concurrent review of hospital care. Presently there is little focus by these firms on the utilization of outpatient care.

In these types of systems, the reviewer has been empowered to authorize payment for reviewed care, but they generally are limited to services explicitly covered by the benefit plan. Most reviewer firms do not have the authority to "flex the benefit plan." Although some case management may be offered, it is minimal, such as letting the treating facility or physician know about some other resource available in their community. The system does not directly offer alternative services nor provide access to a contracted network of providers.

Generally, such firms assume no financial risk. The service providers, on the other hand, do stand the risk of not receiving payment if the reviewer determines that initial or ongoing care is not needed and the provider goes ahead and provides the treatment.

HEALTH MAINTENANCE ORGANIZATIONS (HMOs)

HMOs are the most common form of managed care system. Although varying in structure, the most essential feature is that comprehensive health care services are provided on a prepaid, capitated fee basis. That is, a provider system accepts so many dollars per member per month in return for guaranteeing all the care necessary within the limits of the benefit plan.

The person covered by an HMO, the enrollee, has an assigned primary care physician who serves as the gatekeeper for their entry into any further care. The gatekeeper assesses what is needed and authorizes any referrals to an appropriate specialist provider. Therefore, the primary physician has the case management responsibility within the HMO.

The cost of any care incurred outside of the HMO is generally not reimbursed unless the enrollee was outside the geographical area covered by the HMO and it was an emergency procedure. However, a recent trend noted in the HMO industry is to reimburse enrollees for the cost of care incurred outside the HMO, but at a reduced rate.

There are two primary types of HMOs: the staff model and the independent practice association (IPA) model. In the staff model, all the treatment personnel are salaried employees of the HMO and work out of facilities owned by the HMO. In the IPA model, the HMO contracts with independent providers from the local community to treat members of the HMO within their private offices and clinics, retaining their own practice as an independent practitioner.

Methods of reimbursement for providers can vary within each of the different models. In the staff model, the primary providers are salaried by the HMO, but the specialists to whom the HMO refers patients may be paid on the basis of a discounted fee-for-service or paid a percentage of a "risk-pool" that represents the difference between the premiums paid by the employers and enrollees and the costs of providing the care that is used. In the IPA model, the professional staff, primary care physicians, specialists, and other facilities, hospitals, and clinics may be paid on a capitated basis, a percent of premium basis, a "per case or episode" basis, or, for some, a discounted fee-for-service basis. In addition to this compensation, some providers can earn incentive payments based upon savings from the "risk pool." More recently there has been some efforts to allocate incentives based upon quality of care indicators rather than on financial savings alone.

In summary, the HMO provides a full array of health care services that is covered by a capitated payment, putting the HMO at risk for the cost of the care it provides. Care is case-managed and authorized by the primary care physician, who may or may not share the risk of the HMO but who has incentives to keep the cost of care at a minimum.

PREFERRED PROVIDER ORGANIZATION (PPO)

A preferred provider organization is a network of providers that collectively provide comprehensive health care coverage or an array of specialty care, such as mental health and substance abuse care (Cowan, 1984). The providers contract with a PPO administrator to provide specified types of care within the limits of the employee benefit plan as negotiated between the PPO administrator and the employer/payor. Members of the PPO are independent providers and can include hospitals, group practices, private individual providers, and private agencies. Providers are invited to join the network for one or more different reasons: reputation for quality, geographical location, provision of a necessary specialty service or procedure, or the ability to provide a comprehensive range of subspecialty services.

The PPO administrator, usually a separate managed care corporation or insurance company, undertakes to market the services of the network to employers. In some cases a coalition of employers may develop their own PPO and hire a managed care company to manage it.

31

Providers in a PPO contract to be paid on a discounted fee-for-service basis, *after* services are rendered. Their primary risk is that their discount, based on expected volume of new patients, will not compensate for the actual volume of new patients they treat by virtue of being a member of the PPO network. In addition to addressing the issues of discounted fees and patient volume, most PPO contracts also include specific references regarding the providers' obligations to abide by specific review and authorization mechanisms.

A network of providers alone does not constitute a managed care system, but rather the provider or service component of that system. It becomes a managed care program when it adds utilization review or case management, and when it has the power to authorize payment when covered beneficiaries receive authorized care. These are the functions carried out by the PPO administrator.

Under most circumstances the PPO administrator is at some collective risk for the aggregate cost of the care provided, having been paid a premium by the employer for providing all necessary services to a defined population. In some cases, however, the employer may have paid a fee to the PPO only in order to have access to the "quality at a discount" represented by the PPO network of providers.

COMMUNITY MENTAL HEALTH CENTERS (CMHCs)

Some community mental health centers could fit within our definition of a specialty managed care system. The original concept of the CMHC was a well-managed system offering comprehensive services to a defined population or community. But the financial mechanisms were not appropriate to this mandate, and, as centers developed, the comprehensive mandate changed to focus on those specialized patient groups with serious and prolonged mental illness. However, this focus did require that case management systems become a central part of the CMHC service delivery system.

Because of their limited resources, utilization review programs were instituted by CMHCs to assure that care was provided efficiently. Beyond this level of control, some CMHCs have been able to arrange for either private or public funding on a capitated basis. These centers then assume the financial risk of providing all needed care to a specific population. In these centers, utilization review and case management are critical elements in providing quality services in an efficient manner.

HOW CMHCs CAN BECOME
INVOLVED IN MANAGED CARE SYSTEMS

As just described, some CMHCs are already in the managed care business. The emergence of managed care has opened the door to a new opportunity for mental health centers to enter a sector of the market that can offer a substantial source of new revenues, especially by becoming more involved in the for-profit sector. In this section we review some factors that may make it difficult for some centers to get involved with managed care. These are presented with the hope that they will stimulate centers to examine the potential problems they might face when exploring the possibilities presented by a managed care system.

FACTORS LIMITING CMHC
PARTICIPATION IN MANAGED CARE

Factors limiting participation involve both clinical and administrative issues. One concern that would exist for both clinicians and administrators is the apparent conflict between economic factors and the clinical value system. When going financially at-risk, the center must institute further financial controls on clinical services to individual patients. Although center staff are accustomed to financial limits on a programmatic basis, some clinicians may resist such controls on a case-by-case basis. Ultimately, all parts of the center must come to an understanding that care is, always has been, and will continue to be provided within the constraints of limited funding, whether that funding is based on grants from government, fee-for-service reimbursement, or capitated prepayment.

With that truism in mind, the question for administrators and clinicians becomes one of how to provide quality care in the most efficient, effective manner possible. This frame of reference will necessitate a great deal of creativity by center staff, to determine not only how to manage an individual case, but also in deciding how to allocate overall CMHC resources so that effective, less costly alternative services can be developed. If these questions are not faced and answered, centers will inevitably be excluded from this sector of care and will find it more difficult to adequately provide services for the populations they already serve.

Given that PPOs and HMOs are seeking to contract with providers of care who emphasize quality and cost-effectiveness, CMHC clinicians must come to grips with their orientation toward the length of treatment. Many clinicians were trained to do long-term psychotherapy and have great difficulty accepting the efficiency and benefits of brief treatment. Although we cannot attempt to answer the questions raised by this debate, there is substantial evidence on the efficacy of brief treatment (MacKenzie, 1988). It is clear that this is not the treatment of choice for all persons. However, goal-oriented, brief treatment has proven to be effective and *must* be employed if a center is to use its resources efficiently (Kessler, Steinwachs, & Hankin, 1982).

An issue that involves clinicians, especially primary clinicians, is their possible devaluation of case management. The vast majority of professional therapists insist that they do not do case management, and many do not even understand the role and activities carried out by a case manager. Most CMHCs that have adopted "case management systems" for severely disabled, long-term patients, have assigned separate staff persons, generally at a paraprofessional level of expertise, to be case managers. Consequently, case management functions are not seen as truly "professional."

For the sake of efficiency and greater understanding among the members of each treatment team, primary clinicians must get over their hesitancy to participate in case management. They need to understand how case management supports and enhances therapeutic outcomes. There are just too few resources available to allow one segment of our providers to opt out of participating in this critical service.

A final clinical factor that can limit CMHCs' participation is resistance toward utilization review. External evaluation of a provider's or agency's clinical practices can be experienced as threatening. But with the shifts occurring in the general health care industry, providers will not have the option much longer as to whether or not they will become involved in clinical oversight and review. CMHCs need to start training clinicians to actively participate in review systems and see it as part of their clinical planning, rather than viewing it as the specter of an outside, controlling entity.

Certainly some providers have had bad experiences with reviewers. However, as review systems have become more sophisticated, and more highly qualified clinicians are becoming reviewers, it is more appropriate to view the utilization review process as a collegial one. Clearly, this approach will be more productive for both the reviewer and provider, and it will ultimately lead to decision making about the care to be offered that will be most appropriate for the patient.

Finally, there may be hesitancy among agency administrators to enter into a managed care contract. This hesitancy can be due to lack of experience in negotiating contracts and to a lack of expertise within the organization in determining the utilization and cost projections needed to survive the contract negotiation process. Without the clinical and accounting information systems, coupled with the analytical expertise to make these projections, the director can have little confidence that the prices negotiated in the contract will cover costs *and* generate some contribution to the center's general overhead. This lack of systems and analytical ability should be a real concern because the center may be going at some financial risk in the contract. Later sections of this chapter address some of these concerns in a rudimentary fashion. The CMHC director must go beyond this point and invest more energy in learning the basics of cost and utilization projections.

MAKING USE OF EXISTING TECHNOLOGIES

Although many CMHCs may not have the technological sophistication to project utilization by a specific population, they do have long-standing expertise in several areas that makes them well suited to participation in the managed care industry. This expertise includes case management, working with employers through EAPs, and developing alternative care programs.

First, we will examine the expertise that CMHCs have in the area of case management. This function is one that CMHCs have been performing for years with persons with prolonged mental illness. In fact, the case management done by CMHCs could well serve as the model for the case management used by some managed care providers. Many CMHCs have demonstrated the effectiveness of their case management by reducing the utilization of hospital care in the populations they serve. This record is all the more extraordinary because they have done so with the most chronic segment of the mentally ill population. CMHCs should explore ways to sell this expertise to managed care providers who are looking for specialized case management services for mental health and substance abuse problems. Alternatively, CMHCs could use their case management expertise as the basis for de-

35

signing their own managed care system to be marketed to comprehensive health care providers or to purchasers who want to control administrative costs.

CMHCs can market their managed care capacity as an additional service to employers with whom they have an employee assistance contract. The existence of relationships between CMHCs and employers is a ready path for entering into the managed care market. It is likely that employers who care enough about their employees to offer an EAP will also be concerned enough about them to offer a quality mental health and substance abuse benefit. However, as in all aspects of their operations, employers will look to do this in the most efficient manner. Therefore, while offering mental health services to employers, CMHCs should market and emphasize their expertise in case management, the comprehensiveness of their services, and their ability to offer alternatives to hospitalization. Evidence should be presented regarding the center's effectiveness in reducing the use of hospitalization, and by inference, the cost savings that could be realized by using the center to manage the company's entire mental health benefit.

Finally, and perhaps most importantly, CMHCs should make use of their expertise in innovation by promoting existing alternatives to hospital care as well as developing additional alternatives that meet the needs of high utilization populations (e.g., adolescent substance abusers). Many centers have been willing to take risks by developing these alternative programs, and to the extent that they are available, they will be purchased by managed care providers and others who desire effective, less costly alternatives. This strategy represents a potential source of new revenues for centers interested in broadening their base of financial support. In addition, it offers staff the option to work in a greater variety of program settings to enhance the professional opportunities offered by the CMHC. As staff retention becomes a concern, these options will be helpful in maintaining a loyal, experienced staff.

BECOMING A PART OF THE MANAGED CARE INDUSTRY

In this section we will examine more specifically the ways in which CMHCs can become involved in managed care. In doing so, it is impossible to exhaust all of the alternatives. The permutations in terms of systems of providers, benefit design, statutory regulations, and financial arrangements are numerous and in a state of constant flux. Therefore, it is up to the imagination of those involved to come up with creative solutions to designing a particular managed care system for a local community.

Perhaps the most straightforward way to become involved in managed care is for the CMHC to develop its own system of marketing to purchasers. The primary challenge will be to determine how to package and price these services to meet the specific needs of the payors and purchasers of health care. This task is similar to that faced by centers in packaging their EAPs. The greatest difficulty here is in pricing the service in a way that is attractive to the buyer and yields a profit. Most managed care services also require effort and information to accurately project utilization so that the subsequent price is correctly derived.

For centers that do not already have the basic components of a managed care system described earlier, the first task will be to develop the missing elements. In doing this, it would make sense to survey local purchasers of care to learn what direct treatment services are needed, especially alternative settings for specific populations. By developing services that will meet the needs of high utilization groups, the managed care product offered will be more attractive to the purchaser and will position the center to provide additional services in the future for other high utilization groups.

If the CMHC is not interested in independently developing and marketing its own managed care system, it could subcontract with an HMO or PPO to be a specialty provider. In either situation, the CMHC could seek to provide all required mental health services or to be the provider of specific services. The greatest concern in making this type of arrangement is negotiating the contract to become a part of the managed care system.

Negotiating a Managed Care Contract - Financial Concerns. Whether negotiating with an HMO or a PPO, the CMHC director needs to have a clear understanding of the actual fixed and variable costs of the various CMHC services that will be the focus of the contract. The director also needs to know the percentage of each service's volume, costs, and earned revenues relative to the center's total mix of services. Furthermore, depending on the type of "unit" being negotiated, the CMHC needs to have some understanding of the utilization patterns of the various services as a function of the characteristics of the user population.

There are risks and benefits to be considered by each party to the negotiation. One of the easiest ways to describe those risks from the provider's viewpoint is to review how they vary as a function of the type of "unit of service" or "unit of payment" being considered (Ernst & Whinney, 1986).

1. The least risk for a provider is to give a "percentage discount" off their usual charge for a procedure or unit. In this case the degree of risk is directly related to the final "volume" of the particular service units provided and the variable cost per unit or procedure.
2. The next greatest degree of risk may be assumed when negotiating "per diem" units. Hospitals and day programs can aggregate all ancillary services usually provided to a patient to determine an average, all-inclusive fixed daily rate for any individual patient. The provider is then at risk to the extent that he or she can properly estimate average utilization of services for each individual patient and project actual future costs. If actual per-patient ancillary utilization varies, or costs change, then the provider might not cover its costs.
3. Risks increase further when negotiating "per case" rates of payment. In such agreements care is contracted on the basis of some classification of patients, similar to the Diagnosis Related Groups (DRGs) used in general medical care. The classification, however, need not be limited to diagnostic criteria. For example, there may be a higher payment for "children and adolescents" than for "adult" cases. The price to be paid to the provider is presumably based on the average per case for that particular classification. In addition to the risks involved with per diem rates, this method places the provider at risk when the length of care or total volume of services per patient exceeds the average.
4. Further risks are inherent in "per capita" contracts. In this type of contract, the provider agrees to offer all needed services of a specified type to a specific population group in return for a periodic fixed payment that is made for each member of the group. This type of contract adds to all of the previous risks the additional risk of predicting the frequency of use of services by the members of the population. If it exceeds the expected utilization for that type of population, the provider will not cover its costs.

5. The greatest risk exists when the provider is asked to accept a "percent of premium." This contract is similar to a capitation arrangement, but the payment is based on a percentage of the premiums for the specified population. Therefore, in addition to the previous risks, this type of contract puts the provider at risk on an actuarial basis. If the actuarial assumptions that were used to determine the premium are not correct, then the premium will not cover all services needed and the percentage received by the provider will not be sufficient to cover the needs of the entire population. Furthermore, if the provider invests capital to cover the population, but the HMO/insurer does not sell a sufficient number of contracts to employers, then the investment could be lost.

Although all of these types of risk contracts are possible, the most frequently used by PPOs are discounted charges and per diem discounts, while HMOs will use these two in addition to per-capita contracts.

In a PPO arrangement, the managed care company will negotiate with "preferred" individual and institutional providers for discounted rates or fees to be charged for specified procedures or units of care. The incentive to the provider is the expectation of an increase in the volume of referred patients to take up unused treatment capacity and make further contributions to fixed overhead expenses. The provider assumes the risk that these reduced charges will not cover his or her full fixed and variable expenses.

As in the case of a PPO agreement, in an HMO negotiation the CMHC may be asked to agree to negotiated discounts. Alternatively, the CMHC might be asked to accept a prepaid amount per subscriber and assume the entire risk for certain services, within the limits set by the benefit plan.

Even though it is easy to focus on potential risks in contracting, one must keep in mind the positive consequences. For example, when a provider is asked to accept discounted charges, he or she is usually asked to do so on the basis of receiving a significant volume of business *and* that payment will be made rapidly following the provision of care. In fact, in any type of risk contract, there is always the probability that utilization or costs will be less than projected, in which case the provider stands to make an even greater than expected profit.

To illustrate some of the relationships of volume to discounts, Table 1 (p. 41) presents a hypothetical case where a CMHC's current financial situation is contrasted with three possible scenarios when they contract with a managed care company for the services of their XYZ Program. The three scenarios represent different levels of increased volume, coupled with different levels of discounts for Program XYZ's services.

Note that Program XYZ represents only 20% of the CMHC's total revenue. We are assuming that the new PPO agreement will bring in new volume and revenues *without displacing existing levels of services and revenues*. In other words, the CMHC is selling some slack resources or unused capacity. In some cases this type of assumption is not warranted and the calculations would have to reflect some decreases in current revenue sources if it was necessary to divert existing resources to the new PPO-referred patients.

The new PPO revenues in each of the three scenarios will vary as a function of the discount *and* the volume. Of course, the best relative outcome for the CMHC is Scenario A, where they achieve a 20% volume increase with only a 10% discount. Scenario B produces the relatively poorest outcome but still a positive one.

Negative outcomes are also possible in cases where a deep discount is offered, the new volume displaces old volume, but not enough total volume is realized to offset the discount given. Negotiated discounts should not be so great that they cause revenues to fall below the increase in variable expenses caused by the increase in volume. One possible negotiating strategy to take is to offer a smaller discount for the first increment in volume, and larger discounts for greater increments in volume thereafter. Volume and discount trade-offs become even more critical when they are offered for the services that constitute the largest share of the CMHC's total revenue.

The foregoing discussion also assumes that there is sufficient, unused "fixed capacity" to absorb the increased volume. If additional fixed costs must be incurred in order to accept the contract, the nature of the price and volume negotiations would change accordingly. On the other hand, if there is relatively substantial unused but fixed program capacity and costs, variable costs and volume issues may be irrelevant. Any increases in volume and revenues are simply an added benefit.

The center director must also take into account the potential for a loss in *current program* volume if a contract is *not* negotiat-

TABLE 1: EFFECT OF PPO DISCOUNT AND VOLUME
EXPECTATIONS FOR A PROGRAM
ON THE CENTER'S TOTAL PROFITS

Total Center Revenues	$5,000,000
Total Center Expenses	$4,700,000
Total "Profit"	$300,000
Total "Profit" Margin	6.00%
Program XYZ's Revenues	$1,000,000
Program XYZ's Expenses	$900,000
Variable Expenses	$400,000
Fixed Expenses	$500,000
Profit	$100,000
Profit Margin	10%

XYZ Program's Contribution to:

1. Center's Revenues	20%
2. Center's Expenses	19%
3. Center's Profits	33%

	Scenario A	Scenario B	Scenario C
Following a PPO Agreement:			
Volume Increase	20%	10%	20%
(Totally New Business)			
Negotiated Discount	10%	10%	20%
Program XYZ's Revenues:			
From Non-PPO Sources	$1,000,000	$1,000,000	$1,000,000
From PPO (Discounted)	$180,000	$90,000	$160,000
Variable Expenses	$480,000	$440,000	$480,000
Fixed Expenses	$500,000	$500,000	$500,000
Adjusted "XYZ" Profits	$200,000	$150,000	$180,000
Change in "XYZ" Profits	$100,000	$50,000	$80,000
Total Center Profits	$400,000	$350,000	$380,000
Change from Base	33.33%	16.67%	26.67%

ed. That is, some of the CMHC's current business may be lost if the HMO or PPO has the ability to steer referrals away from the CMHC. Conversely, the CMHC should be reasonably sure that any volume increases are ones they would not get otherwise without signing the contract.

The final example will illustrate some of the financial benefits that a managed care contract can provide by virtue of such functions as preassessing each patient's condition, triaging patients to improve scheduling and "show-rates," and improving speed of payment and net collection rates. Table 2 (p. 44-45) illustrates two different outpatient programs, before and after receiving a PPO contract. Both programs are identical in two respects, total expenses and number of full-time equivalent (FTE) clinical staff. As illustrated in Table 2, there are some relative differences between them in how well they are managed on such key indicators as (a) productivity standards for clinical staff, (b) percentage of capacity scheduled for visits, (c) average rate of appointments kept by patients, and (d) average rate of billed charges actually collected.

These two programs are described in the first and third columns of numbers as if they had no PPO contracts. The second and fourth columns depict the possible effects of *identical* PPO contracts, yielding an increased volume of 30%, based on a discount of 15%. In both programs the PPO volume increases are assumed to displace non-PPO volume, that is, holding total therapy hours available constant.

By examining the details in Table 2, the reader can see that the PPO contract has helped both programs. Although the absolute financial gain is greater for the poorly managed Program 1, going from a $26,113 loss to a $4,310 gain, Program 2's relative improvement from $39,967 to $65,885 makes its efficiency even greater (e.g., cost per therapy hour, net profit per therapy hour, and return on the $180,000 expenses investment). These relative effects are related to *nonfinancial factors* that potentially derive from involvement with a managed care system.

Specifically, managed care patients are more likely to be efficiently scheduled, have higher rates of keeping their appointments, and lead to improved net collections because the contract guarantees the payment of the agreed-upon rate. Sliding fee adjustments are not applicable. Although Table 2 does not illustrate the benefit of *faster* payment, there is an additional cash flow advantage to being paid promptly. Furthermore, Table 2 does not show the effect on revenues from billing the patient for any applicable copayments. Of course, not every managed care contract may yield each or any of the nonfinancial benefits. In any case, it is the responsibility of the CMHC director to look for such benefits during the negotiation process.

Offsetting these advantages are the additional costs involved with compliance with contract requirements such as the staff time necessary for clinical review by the managed care firm. In our experience, however, such staff time is negligible relative to total staff time and therefore does not add appreciably to the fixed costs of care.

In addition to these specific price and volume concerns, there are a few other financial issues that will typically arise in contract negotiations. One item will cover the provider's right to balance bill the patient for copayments as spelled out by the insurance benefit plan. There may also be limits to billing the patient for services that were not authorized by the reviewer or for services not covered by the benefit plan. Usually the provider may bill the patient for these services only if the patient agrees in writing to receive these services *prior* to their being provided. In most cases the provider will be required to absorb the costs of reviews and any costs related to the request for medical records. In some circumstances, however, the provider may successfully negotiate for reimbursement of these costs.

The final financial issues will involve the speed of payment the provider can expect following the submission of a valid claim and procedures for resolving claims disputes.

Negotiating a Contract - Clinical and Administrative Issues.
The CMHC director should expect to negotiate a number of issues related to general administrative and clinical review processes inherent in a managed care contract. These issues involve the obligations and rights of the provider and the obligations and rights of the managed care company.

The provider should expect to receive details of the review process in a "Provider Review Manual." This manual will spell out such details as the benefit plan and the definition of covered services and exclusions, procedures for determining beneficiary eligibility and levels of coverage, clinical criteria to be used in making service authorizations, procedures to follow in making referrals of patients, and the number to call if there are questions regarding claims payment.

The provider will be obligated to maintain some minimum level of malpractice insurance, make arrangements for the emer-

TABLE 2: EFFECTS OF IDENTICAL PPO CONTRACTS ON TWO IDENTICALLY SIZED OUTPATIENT PROGRAMS, EACH OF WHICH IS DIFFERENTLY MANAGED
(PPO Volume Increase = 30% and PPO Discount = 15%)

Outpatient Program	Program 1		Program 2	
	Before PPO	With PPO	Before PPO	With PPO
Total Expenses	$180,000.00	$180,000.00	$180,000.00	$180,000.00
FTE Clinical Staff	4	4	4	4
Productivity Standard	50%	50%	50%	60%
Available Hours	4160	4160	4992	4992
For Non-PPO Clients	4160	2912	4992	3494
For PPO Clients	NA	1248	NA	1498
Budgeted Cost/Hour	$43.27	$43.27	$36.06	$36.06
Scheduling Efficiency				
For Non-PPO Clients	85%	85%	90%	90%
For PPO Clients	NA	95%	NA	95%
Hours Scheduled				
For Non-PPO Clients	3536	2475	4493	3145
For PPO Clients	NA	1186	NA	1423
Show-Rate Efficiency				
For Non-PPO Clients	80%	80%	85%	85%
For PPO Clients	NA	95%	NA	95%
Therapy Hours Provided				
For Non-PPO Clients	2829	1980	3819	2673
For PPO Clients	NA	1126	NA	1352

Average Charge/Hour				
For Non-PPO Clients	$80.00	$80.00	$80.00	$80.00
For PPO Clients	NA	$68.00	NA	$68.00
Sliding Scale Adjustment				
For Non-PPO Clients	20%	20%	20%	20%
For PPO Clients	NA	None	NA	None
Net Charge/Hour				
For Non-PPO Clients	$64.00	$64.00	$64.00	$64.00
For PPO Clients	NA	$68.00	NA	$68.00
Average Collection Rate				
For Non-PPO Clients	85%	85%	90%	90%
For PPO Clients	NA	100%	NA	100%
Dollars Collected/Hour				
For Non-PPO Clients	$54.40	$54.40	$57.60	$57.60
For PPO Clients	NA	$68.00	NA	$68.00
TOTAL COLLECTIONS	$153,887.00	$184,310.00	$219,967.00	$245,885.00
Performance Indicators				
Revenue/Therapy Hour	$54.40	$59.33	$57.60	$61.09
Cost/Therapy Hour	$63.63	$57.94	$47.13	$44.72
Profit (Loss)/Hour	($9.23)	$1.39	$10.47	$16.37
Total Profit (Loss)	($26,113.00)	$4,310.00	$39,967.00	$65,885.00
Change in Profit or Loss		$30,424.00		$25,917.00
Return on Investment	-14.51%	2.39%	22.20%	36.60%

gency availability of some services, if applicable, and in some cases provide for the coverage of weekends and evening hours. Furthermore, the provider is likely to be required to notify the managed care company of any incidents that would compromise its ability to provide the contracted services, such as a fire or natural disaster, loss of equipment or personnel, or loss of certification or licensure. In addition to maintaining appropriate licenses and certifications, the provider organization may be required to assure that their employees maintain appropriate personal and professional licenses. The provider's rights to subcontract or assign the contract will also be specified.

Providers may be limited in their rights to communicate directly with the benefit manager of the patient's employer, being required instead to handle disputes directly with the managed care company. There may also be some limits on the provider in how he or she discusses with the patient any review decisions made by the managed care company.

The contract may cover the provider's rights to use the managed care company's name in any advertising or promotional activities. Conversely, the managed care company's obligations or limits to using the provider's name should also be specified. In some cases the employer or insurer will want to list the preferred providers' names, addresses, and specialties in booklets distributed to employees.

Contracts will define the scope of the managed care company's rights to review the patient's medical records. Most limitations will be based on local, state, and federal statutes governing access to psychiatric and substance abuse records.

Mechanisms for resolving disputes and remedies for breach of contract should be spelled out. Generally there are clauses addressing the mutual indemnification of the parties in circumstances of lawsuits in connection with the agreement. Finally, the contract should spell out conditions affecting the termination of the contract, including the rights of either party to end the contract with or without cause. Termination issues generally address the reasons for termination, such as illegal or fraudulent conduct, the methods and timing of notification, and the obligations of the provider to responsibly conclude the treatment of the patients still in treatment at time of termination, or arrange for their transfer in cooperation with the managed care company. In turn, the managed care company will be obligated to pay for agreed-upon services rendered to such patients, if any, beyond the termination date.

SUMMARY

In order to address the growing concerns of employers and insurers regarding the cost and quality of health care, managed care systems in the form of HMOs and PPOs will become increasingly prevalent. Specialized systems for managing mental health and substance abuse benefits will also expand parallel to, or as an inherent part of, these larger health care systems. Although community mental health centers have many reasons to be hopeful that they can participate in this growing market, their participation will depend on many factors, including the quality of the center's services and the capabilities of its administrative and management systems.

Center administrators and clinical staff should examine their current services and management capabilities and assess their readiness to enter into managed care systems, either as a provider for other managed care companies or as a managed care company themselves. Although there are some complex financial, legal, and clinical concerns, the potential for growth and profitability is excellent. Success, in turn, can result in improvements and enhancements for the core mission of the center, the care of the general population, and those most seriously in need of services.

Anthony Broskowski, PhD, is Director of Health Care Research and Evaluation for the Prudential Insurance Company. Prior to this position, he served as Senior Vice President and Senior Analyst at Preferred Health Care, Ltd. which specializes in mental health case management. From 1977 to 1986 he served as the Executive Director of Northside Centers in Tampa, Florida, where he developed a comprehensive and innovative series of alternative mental health programs for adults and children. Dr. Broskowski may be contacted at Prudential Insurance Company, HCORD, Stop 410, 56 N. Livingston Avenue, Roseland, NJ 07068.

Edward Marks, PhD, is a licensed psychologist who is currently Executive Director of United Behavioral Systems, Georgia, a division of a national managed care company in Atlanta, Georgia. Prior to this, Dr. Marks was responsible for development of managed mental health care programs for a major telecommunications company, and had been Executive Director of a comprehensive community mental health center. He can be contacted at United Behavioral Systems, Georgia, 3390 Peachtree Road, N.E., Suite 700, Atlanta, GA 30326.

REFERENCES

Alt, S. (1988). Xerox spends money to save money on mental health care. *Contract Healthcare*, pp. 39-40.

Bagby, N., & Sullivan, S. (1986). *Buying Smart: Business Strategies for Managing Health Care Costs*. Washington, DC: American Enterprise Institute.

Bridwell, D., Collins, J., & Levine, D. (1988). A quiet revolution: The movement of EAPs to managed care. *EAP Digest, 8*, 27-30.

Brightbill, T. (1988). Mental health firms offer more care for less cost. *Contract Healthcare*, pp. 9-11.

Cowan, D. (1984). *Preferred Provider Organizations*. Rockville, MD: Aspen Systems Corp.

Ernst & Whinney (Consulting Firm). (1986). *Health Care Risk Contracting* (E & W Number J58654). New York: Author.

Feldstein, P., Wickizer, T., & Wheeler, J. (1988). Private cost containment: The effects of utilization review programs on health care use and expenditures. *New England Journal of Medicine, 318,* 1310-1314.

Fine, M. (1988). Managing mental health care greatly lowers costs. *Managed Care Outlook, 1,* 3-4.

Foster-Higgins (Consulting Firm). (1989). *Health Care Benefits Survey, 1988*. Princeton, NJ: Author.

Frank, R., & Kamlet, M. (1985). Direct costs and expenditures for mental health care in the United States in 1980. *Hospital and Community Psychiatry, 36,* 165-168.

Goldstein, J., & Horgan, C. (1988). Inpatient and outpatient psychiatric services: Substitutes or complements? *Hospital and Community Psychiatry, 39,* 632-636.

Herzlinger, R., & Calkins, D. (1986). How companies tackle health care costs: Part III. *Harvard Business Review, 64,* 70-80.

Kessler, L., Steinwachs, D., & Hankin, J. (1982). Episodes of psychiatric care and medical utilization. *Medical Care, 20,* 1209-1221.

Kiesler, C. (1982). Public and professional myths about mental hospitalization: An empirical reassessment of policy-related beliefs. *American Psychologist, 37,* 1323-1339.

Kiesler, C., & Sibulkin, A. (1987). *Mental Hospitalization: Myths and Facts about a National Crisis*. Newbury Park, CA: Sage.

MacKenzie, K. (1988). Recent developments in brief psycho-therapy. *Hospital and Community Psychiatry, 39,* 742-752.

Mechanic, D. (1985). Cost containment and the quality of medical care: Rationing strategies in an era of constrained resources. *Milbank Memorial Fund Quarterly: Health and Society, 63,* 453-475.

Melnick, S., & Lyter, L. (1987). The negative impacts of increased concurrent review of psychiatric inpatient care. *Hospital and Community Psychiatry, 38,* 300-302.

Miller, W., & Hester R. (1986). Inpatient alcoholism treatment: Who benefits? *American Psychologist, 41,* 794-805.

Milstein, A., Oehm, M., & Alpert, G. (1987). Gauging the performance of utilization review. *Business and Health, 4,* 10-12.

National Association of Private Psychiatric Hospitals. (1988). *Ensuring Good Psychiatric Benefits.* Washington, DC: Author.

Steffen, G. (1988). Quality medical care. *Journal of the American Medical Association, 260,* 56-61.

Trauner, J. (1987). The next generation of utilization review. *Business and Health, 4,* 14-16.

Wallace, C. (1987). Employers turning to managed care to control their psychiatric care costs. *Modern Healthcare, July,* 82-84.

3

The "Private" Community Mental Health Organization

Morris L. Eaddy

Today's private, nonprofit community mental health organization (CMHO) is undergoing transformation at an extremely rapid rate due to profound changes occurring in the nation's entire health care industry. Community mental health is now a substantial part of the health care industry and shares many of the same stresses and opportunities that occur during times of dynamic change. At no time in the relatively brief history of community mental health has the job of CMHO management been so frustrating, so fascinating, so stressful, so challenging, and so potentially gratifying.

RECENT CHANGES
IN CMHO MANAGEMENT

As Neeley and Ray (1986b) have pointed out, in recent years there have been dramatic changes in the market management, operation management, financial management, and clinical management of CMHOs. They note that, from a market standpoint, there has been movement from a government-sponsored service delivery system (e.g., the 12 federally mandated services) to the current customer-driven service delivery system and a future payor-driven service delivery system.

Federal funding has been drastically reduced, and state funding has failed to keep pace with inflation. Service demands, however, have increased as have the costs of doing business. New funding, therefore, has been sought from a variety of non-governmental sources. Fee income has become of major importance. Private, nonprofit CMHOs are rapidly learning how to perform financial feasibility studies and marketing analyses, and they see the importance of strategic planning and corporate configuration. A job description for the chief executive officer (CEO) of a modern-day CMHO should include, along with the traditional requisites, general knowledge of quality assurance and risk management, how to secure venture capital, predicting return on investment, utilization review, productivity management, marketing, preserving market share, how to secure managed care contracts, personnel management, and other management skills not required when CMHOs were primarily financed with governmental funds.

From the standpoint of operations management, Neeley and Ray (1986b) describe a transition from a purely clinical orientation, with informal structures developed in a regulated environment, to an orientation that focuses on marketing, quality control, and adaptability to the frequent changes necessary in an increasingly competitive marketplace.

They also describe significant changes in financial management affecting private, nonprofit CMHOs attempting to position themselves in the mainstream of the health care marketplace at a time when alternative systems of health service delivery are rapidly emerging.

CMHOs must take a hard look at cost controls and developing profit centers. They must often struggle to maintain market share as competition for the mental health dollar intensifies. Maintaining market share often requires redefining the mission of the CMHO, structuring certain services to appeal to middle- and high-income clients, and devoting substantial resources to marketing. Proprietary hospitals and other for-profit corporations are investing heavily not only in inpatient but also in residential treatment, outpatient treatment, and day or evening treatment programs. These for-profit corporations have the potential of capturing a significant portion of the market that has historically been served by the nonprofit CMHO.

Clinical management is shifting from traditional staffing practices to a human resource management model which includes outside review of clinical services, employment of "payor-eligible" practitioners, contingent compensation of clinicians, and a strong emphasis upon quality assurance and conservative resource utilization.

THE INCREASED NEED FOR SERVICES

Provision of mental health and substance abuse services has become big business in this country. The private, nonprofit CMHO is only one of an increasing number of providers. Health Maintenance Organizations (HMOs), Preferred Provider Organizations (PPOs), and Employee Assistance Programs (EAPs) exist throughout the nation and strongly influence the future of the community mental health and substance abuse programs. Mental health has become a big business because the need for services is so great, the stigma for receiving services has lessened somewhat, and third-party reimbursement for services is growing as society recognizes that treatment of mental health and substance abuse problems is a significant health issue that must be addressed.

This need for services is reflected in National Institute of Mental Health statistics (NIMH; 1988) indicating that approximately one in five adult Americans suffers from at least one disorder classified as psychiatric, including substance abuse. Ernst and Whinney (1987) suggest that the stigma associated with receiving services has been reduced to "a marked increase in the marketing of mental health services directly to the ultimate consumer" (p. 12). They also note, with regard to increased availability of third-party reimbursement, that coverage for mental health and substance abuse treatment services is becoming standard for most medium- to large-size corporations:

In return for increased coverage plans, business and industry, government programs, and insurance companies will require increased documentation of treatment effectiveness, greater emphasis on lower cost outpatient programs, and enhanced utilization review efforts by providers to offset their unfamiliarity with these services, the lack of widely accepted treatment methodologies, and concerns with cost control. (Ernst & Whinney, 1987, p. 25)

They give the following examples of sound business reasons for corporate America to include mental health and substance abuse coverage:

Kennecott Copper Company's "Insight" counseling program reports a 53 percent reduction in absenteeism and 55 percent hospital/surgical/medical reductions.

Group Health Association (a Washington, D.C. health maintenance organization) reports that users of mental health counseling benefits reduced their nonpsychiatric physician benefits by 30.7 percent and lab/x-ray services by 29.8 percent.

General Motors' alcoholism program reports a 49 percent reduction in lost work hours and a 29 percent reduction in disability costs.

In summary, mental health services are fast becoming a payor-driven system with a major focus on cost-containment and quality assurance control. (Ernst & Whinney, 1987, p. 25)

COMPETITIVE FINANCIAL PLANNING

The traditional private, nonprofit CMHO is finding that it is no longer possible to chart a successful future on governmental funding, either state or federal. Continued dependence on primarily state or federal funding will restrict the service mission to only those people who are designated as high-priority clients by state or federal legislation. If a reasonable range of services is to be provided to other clients, funding must be obtained from other sources, and increasing first- and third-party fee income must become an important goal.

As managers of many nonprofit corporations have learned, sometimes in a painful way, if a "nonprofit" corporation does not produce a reasonable amount of income in excess of expenses (i.e., "profit"), the corporation will eventually cease to exist or will be forced to severely restrict its mission (Perry, 1987). The nonprofit status insures that net income is not distributed to members of the corporation or employees but is used to further the purpose and mission of the corporation. Like any business, however, the nonprofit corporation must secure surplus income for a number of legitimate and important purposes:

- Depreciation - to replace equipment and repair facilities.
- Construction of new facilities.
- Renovation of older facilities to accommodate current service needs.

- Renovation of facilities required to meet more exacting fire and safety standards; comply with licensing requirements; meet accreditation criteria required by the Joint Commission on Accreditation of Healthcare Organizations (JCAHO), the Commission on Accreditation of Rehabilitation Facilities (CARF), or similar accrediting organizations.
- Compensation - well-qualified professionals are required to insure quality services. This is as true in nonprofit corporations as it is in for-profit corporations. Excess discretionary revenue makes it possible for the nonprofit corporation to successfully compete in recruiting well-qualified staff. This helps reduce the high turnover rate of professional staff experienced by many underfunded nonprofits.
- Growth - many important mental health and substance abuse services are needed in any community. To fulfill its corporate purpose for existence, increased and improved services must be an important part of the organization's strategic plan. Often this can only be accomplished through additional discretionary income.
- Cash flow - a reasonable cash flow reserve is required to insure that expenses can be met on a timely basis.
- Audit payback reserve - financial resources must be available for paybacks required from time to time due to disallowances by third-party payors. As nonprofit CMHOs obtain increased income from insurance companies, HMOs, Medicare, Medicaid, and CHAMPUS, the possibility of some charges being disallowed requires that a reserve account be established for payback purposes.

Nonprofits in the mental health field are aware of the many changes occurring, but many are still struggling with the organizational transformation necessary to enable them to continue successful operation.

Although many problems will be involved in this transformation, a major problem that must be directly addressed is that some states may not encourage the necessary changes in operation and, in fact, may place obstacles in the way of implementing sound business practices. There is a question that is sometimes spoken and often implied through rules, regulations, and attitudes: "You are supposed to be nonprofit, so how can you defend a year-end revenue surplus?" This question discloses a frightening lack of understanding concerning the financial realities of operating a sound business. It must be dealt with through improved communication and understanding of sound business principles if the nonprofit CMHO, dependent to any significant extent upon governmental contracts, is to be fiscally sound and able to continue effective operation.

To remain a viable provider in the mental health care market, nonprofit CMHOs must realistically view what the near future holds in store. According to Kipp (1987):

> ... Industry analysts fully expect that before long, nearly 90% of the commercially insured patients in this country will move into the health-care system through some kind of managed care plan. And I firmly believe that the same thing is going to happen with governmentally insured patients. Some states are already contracting out the Medicaid population to managed care plans, and the federal government continues to make a strong push to move Medicare patients into other managed care arrangements as well. (pp. 27-28)

He further states:

> Both general hospitals and private psychiatric facilities are "discovering" the continuum of care and vertically integrating so as to capture market share from both *private* and *public* pay sources. Some classic long-stay psychiatric hospitals are vertically integrating and running both day treatment and outpatient levels of care. (p. 28)

Also:

> The key point is that everyone else within this picture seems to be picking up community mental health "technology" and, by extension, market share. (p. 28)

And finally:

> Don't underestimate the readiness of the private sector to compete for the traditional role of CMHC's and public agencies. No less than 30 states are actively pursuing *private* contracts for either their institutional systems or their community services. (p. 30)

The importance of a constructive response to increasing competition is reflected in the fact that the Center for Health and Human Resources Policy at Harvard University is joining with the National Council of Community Mental Health Centers to study competition among providers of mental health services.

So, what are the facts? The facts are that all mental health providers are either currently experiencing, or will experience in the near future, increased competition, increased need for managerial flexibility, an increasing influence of managed care systems on health care service delivery, and the need for more sophisticated financial planning. The financial planning of nonprofit CMHOs requires the same level of staff expertise and consultative resources as now utilized by the for-profit sector. The nonprofits must develop the means to obtain easier access to the capital necessary to remain competitive and to permit reasonable growth of services. The Ernst and Whinney (1987) report states:

> In order for mental health providers--including CMHCs--to continue to provide high-quality care to populations most in need will require prudent and creative product/services strategies focused on marketing and financial issues. (p. 52)

PLANNING FOR FUTURE GROWTH

In the past several years, some nonprofit CMHOs have taken steps similar to those taken by nonprofit hospitals when these hospitals were initially faced with serious competition from proprietary national hospital chains. In 1977 a number of nonprofit hospitals banded together and formed Voluntary Hospitals of America (VHA). This organization has become extremely successful in assisting its member hospitals in many areas of business such as marketing, consultative services, cost containment services, and cost-reduction through mass purchasing agreements and contracting at preferential or discount rates. VHA can assist nonprofit hospitals in obtaining capital for facilities improvements and new construction. Through development of a captive insurance company, member hospitals have saved millions of dollars in insurance premiums.

A similar organization has recently been formed by a number of nonprofit CMHOs. Mental Health Corporations of America,

Inc. was formed in 1985 to provide its membership benefits similar to those afforded hospitals which are members of VHA.

Even though MHCA is a very young organization, it has already successfully developed a separate professional and general liability insurance company under the provisions of the federal Risk Retention Act. The MHCA membership perceived the growing problem of availability and affordability of professional liability insurance as community mental health centers become the target for a growing number of lawsuits. Development of a "captive" professional and general liability insurance company was a rational response to the need for stable, affordable insurance.

MHCA also provides its membership consultation and information regarding access to capital, new services, marketing, joint ventures, corporate configuration options, new sources of reve nue, and other matters related to improving managerial effectiveness.

In short, the private, nonprofit CMHO must operate with the same managerial and strategic goals as proprietary corporations to successfully carry out the purposes of the nonprofit.

REDEFINING THE CMHO's MISSION

Shea (1986) has stated major requirements for a successful future:

> I think success is going to go to those centers which can convince the paying public that they have the best product for the best price and prove it time and time again. There is nothing that is going to kill you quicker than providing a bad service. Quality of care is going to be an issue along with price and visibility, and those are going to be the things that are going to sustain any system for the next five or ten years.

As might be expected, considering the history of the community mental health "movement," a number of nonprofits are having to struggle to shift gears. They must move from what was historically a quite regulated health care environment to a less regulated one; from relatively stable and predictable governmental revenues to decreased or inadequate governmental funding and the need to develop significant "new" revenue from far less predictable sources; and from being the primary provider of services to having to compete one-on-one with for-profit corporations that are well capitalized and aggressive in their attempts to carve out larger and larger pieces of the mental health marketplace. Nonprofit CMHOs will, as suggested by Ambrose and Lennox (1988), need to carefully position themselves in the ever-changing mental health market.

Some of the nonprofit CMHOs will undoubtedly fail in their attempts to retain their primary identity and mission. Some will try to withdraw to a more narrow mission of dealing almost exclusively with governmental contracts restricted to provision of services to the severely mentally ill and a few other state or federal priority client populations. However, these providers will have to eventually wake up to the fact that even governmental contracts, historically assumed to be "guaranteed" to the nonprofit CMHO, are subject to changes in governmental policy that may in the future include moving from sole-source contracting to competitive bidding.

Any CMHO that believes it will remain a sole-source provider for governmentally funded services is going to be extremely surprised in the next few years. There will be efforts by proprietary groups to enter into that publicly funded market which, when viewed from a national perspective, is an enormous market.

LEARNING FROM THE FOR-PROFIT SECTOR

A growing number of nonprofit CMHOs, however, are making a successful transition. They are learning important lessons from the for-profit sector. Perceived as an opportunity for constructive change rather than being seen as simply a threat to the traditional areas of CMHO service delivery, relationships with the for-profits, which are frequently quite competitive, can help nonprofit CMHOs in many ways. These include improving the quality of services, increasing services to their communities through additional revenue, improving management and strategic planning capabilities, increasing staff compensation to competitive levels, and improving long-term corporate financial stability to insure future growth.

Some nonprofit CMHOs are having successful experience in providing certain services for a "profit," thus allowing these CMHOs to subsidize other essential services that operate at a deficit, to increase services to the indigent, and to insure financial stability and growth. The following services are being operated on a profitable basis by various nonprofit CMHOs:

1. *Short-Term Residential Substance Abuse Treatment.* These treatment programs, offering inpatient treatment, aftercare, and sometimes structured intensive outpatient services, can be profitable if well run and aggressively marketed. They can compete successfully with traditional hospital inpatient substance abuse treatment programs by offering a quite competitive cost-per-treatment episode and gain a respectable market share in the local community.

2. *Long-Term Adolescent Residential Treatment Programs.* A number of CMHOs have been providing these specialized treatment programs for years on a financial break-even basis. With attractive, well-designed facilities, the program could be marketed to full-fee patients.

3. *Consultative Services.* Some CMHOs have been able to produce additional income by providing innovative consultative services to other health care organizations. Areas covered by such services include marketing, board training, strategic planning, performing market analysis for proposed services, and teenage pregnancy prevention. The National Council of Community Mental Health Centers (12300 Twinbrook Parkway, Suite 320, Rockville, MD 20852) can assist in identifying CMHOs that have been especially successful in providing consultative services. These CMHOs can then be contacted and should be able to provide specific information concerning their consultative experiences.

4. *Managed Mental Health and Substance Abuse Treatment Programs Through Capitated Contracts.* A number of larger CMHOs are entering into contracts to provide the mental health and substance abuse treatment services required by managed health care corporations. Capitated contracts provide the CMHO with the potential for substantial profits if the contract is adequately priced and if the CMHO's treatment resources have the capacity to "deliver" the contracted services. There is clear risk in losing money on these contracts if they have not been negotiated with accurate utilization projections. This is certainly an area in which the risks/benefits should be carefully evaluated. It would be wise to consult with CMHOs that have several years' experience in this market before proceeding. It would also be prudent to

obtain specific expert consultation regarding setting appropriate capitation rates.

5. *Outpatient Mental Health and Substance Abuse Services Marketed to Middle- and Upper-Income Level Clients.* In the development of a specialized outpatient service, attention should be given to the need for attractive facilities, strategically located in an area acceptable to such clients. Funds should be budgeted to pay for the marketing that will be necessary and emphasis given to office practices that are "user friendly." The outpatient service can position the CMHO to successfully negotiate managed mental health contracts and effectively triage clients who need residential inpatient hospitalization or partial hospitalization.

6. *Contracts for Vocational Services of Various Types* (e.g., janitorial and grounds maintenance services). Work opportunities for CMHO clients, especially the severely mentally ill and developmentally disabled, are very important aspects of a total treatment program. These services, if properly planned and structured, can become income generators. A number of CMHOs operate vocational programs with budgets of several million dollars. These programs are valuable additions to traditional mental health services, and most CMHOs could expand vocational services by developing realistic business plans for these services. Mental Health Corporations of America (2846-A Remington Green Circle, Tallahassee, FL 32308) can provide information about successful programs. In addition, vocational evaluation and training contracts with private industry councils and state departments of vocational rehabilitation can often be successfully solicited.

7. *Owning and Operating Psychiatric Hospitals.* Hospital inpatient psychiatric services have been a fast-growing market in recent years and, if well managed, can be quite profitable. Although opening a hospital unit requires significant planning and start-up capital, the long-term financial benefits can be sizable. The net revenue from inpatient units can do a great deal to stabilize a CMHO's financial situation. However, with the ever-increasing emphasis on cost containment through managed health care arrangements, hospital inpatient psychiatric services

in many areas of the country are experiencing sharp declines in census. The local market for such services should be carefully considered before a CMHO makes the expensive investment of time and money required to implement such a venture.

8. *Managing Psychiatric Hospitals.* Contracts to manage hospitals are a source of additional income for some CMHOs. The CMHO has extensive clinical and administrative experience in the treatment of mental health patients. A management contract can be profitable and does not require the large commitment of planning and financial resources required of a CMHO that owns and operates its own inpatient unit.

9. *Managing State Owned Mental Health Hospitals.* Although apparently only a few CMHOs are presently contracting with state government to manage state institutions, this is a logical business venture because of the potential of improving continuity of care.

These are only a few of the endeavors that are emerging as nonprofit CMHOs venture into additional legitimate markets. Several decades of community mental health experience have uniquely equipped the CMHO to provide these services in a most cost-effective manner.

However, it is important to keep two factors clearly in mind as any nonprofit CMHO pursues these new ventures:

1. The primary mission of the CMHO to provide services to the acutely and severely mentally ill must be maintained and improved. Additional funding obtained by the CMHO can assist in assuring that this important mission is successfully achieved.

2. The board of directors of the CMHO must be fully informed of "new ventures" and fully supportive of the expanded service mission. This support should be an integral part of the CMHO's long-term strategic plan. Many of the "new ventures" entail a somewhat higher degree of risk than CMHOs have been used to historically. The boards must understand the changes taking place nationally leading to managed health care trends and the

socio-political changes that have made traditional governmental funding much less predictable than in the past.

RESISTANCE TO CMHO
GROWTH IN THE COMMUNITY

Many larger communities have a substantial number of private practitioners, as well as established hospital and residential treatment programs. Resistance in many forms may become evident as a CMHO begins to achieve some success in obtaining a "piece of the private market." Efforts may be made to persuade the CMHO to provide services only to the indigent. There may be protests that the CMHO is "nonprofit" and, therefore, should not engage in services that will produce income in excess of actual expenses. The CMHO must strategically plan for any significant deviation from its mission as perceived by the private practice community, local and state governmental funding sources, and other influential groups. Such groups must be helped to understand the necessity and legitimacy of diversifying CMHO funding sources. Continuation of the public mission depends upon the CMHO's success in achieving a reasonable "client/payor mix."

A similar and perhaps more difficult problem can easily occur in small communities and rural areas where there may only be one or two psychiatrists and the medical community expresses concern about the competition perceived in a new CMHO venture.

The pros and cons of any competitive endeavor or new venture must be carefully weighed, for there are always very real political and organizational issues to be considered whenever a significant change in the scope of the mission of a CMHO is planned.

The for-profit sector, in turn, can learn some valuable lessons from the nonprofit CMHOs, including the necessity for continuity of patient care, the therapeutic value of utilizing least-restrictive treatment modalities, the use of more cost-efficient treatment services by more selective use of hospital inpatient treatment, the use of effective case management, and the societal desirability of earmarking some profits to provide subsidized community services in areas of especially high need.

As stated by Boaz (1988), the service delivery system put in place by nonprofit CMHOs during the past several decades is a model that will be increasingly utilized by the for-profit sector:

Is there a prototype of mental health service delivery already in existence that incorporates the elements of comprehensiveness and continuity of care, crisis intervention, psychological education, the use of community resources, and almost every basic concept associated with effective prepaid mental health care? Yes. The principles of community mental health embody all these elements. CMHCs for years have been obligated to deliver very comprehensive services in the face of fixed, cost-contained budgets to mandated populations. That is what HMOs do. The sources of funding and statutes governing HMO departments of mental health and CMHCs are different, but the concept and procedural techniques learned in the community mental health work can be applied to good advantage in an HMO. (p. 49)

Boaz (1988) further explains:

These agencies (i.e. CMHCs) are becoming aware of the advantages of providing mental health care for HMOs and in many instances are already actively seeking service agreements. (p. 146)

PRIORITIES FOR FUTURE PLANNING

Within the next few years, there will likely be fewer mental health and substance abuse services that will be "guaranteed" to the nonprofit CMHO. CMHOs who have engaged in strategic planning will remain the most viable health care providers.

SUCCESSFUL STRATEGIC PLANNING OF CMHOs

Implement Effective and Efficient Management Practices. This begins with a carefully considered plan for the future of the organization. A clear definition of the organization's mission is essential. The mission should include a commitment to high-quality services, and this implies the need for long-term financial stability of the organization. Management staff, many probably from clinical backgrounds, must be adequately prepared and trained to operate the CMHO as a successful business if the treatment mission is to be achieved. The board of the CMHO should endorse, as board policy, the steps necessary to enable the CMHO to remain a viable health care provider. For example, one board set a clear direction to CMHO management staff by adopting policies stating that:

1. Provision of services to chronically and acutely disturbed persons is a major priority.
2. The corporation shall own, rather than lease, facilities whenever possible.
3. The corporation shall be operated on a sound business basis, utilizing, as necessary, legal, financial, real estate, marketing, or other consultation services required to reach and practice prudent business decisions.
4. Staff are charged with the responsibility of implementing policies adopted by the board.
5. Entrepreneurial, innovative leadership and management of the corporation is encouraged.
6. Staff are directed to position the corporation in such a way as to successfully compete in the general health care market.
7. The corporation's mission shall be broad and flexible to include traditional mental health and alcohol and drug treatment services, as well as other areas of health services to the extent that they (a) are needed in the community, (b) are financially feasible, and (c) can be implemented and managed successfully. In addition, other areas of services or businesses that may result in additional income sources for the betterment of the corporation may be considered. The corporation will aggressively pursue new areas of service or business while maintaining existing quality services.
8. The board will search for ways to improve the corporation's ability to attract and retain talented, experienced staff.
9. The board and staff will work toward greater corporate self-sufficiency and reduced reliance upon governmental funding as the major source of support of the corporation. This includes an emphasis upon diversified funding sources.
10. The board will develop a corporate structure most conducive to achieving the goals of the corporation. This may involve, from time to time, restructuring the organization and/or developing lateral or subsidiary corporations.

11. The board will develop the corporation's capability to attract funding from private donations, foundations, bequests, and other private philanthropic sources.

The specific policy statements of a CMHO may vary considerably from the examples given. However, it is important that clear policy be set so that management staff can work hand in hand with the governing body of the CMHO to achieve the corporate mission. Effective and efficient management practices can then be developed to respond to the policy guidelines.

Engage in High-Quality, Ongoing Training of Staff Who Are Responsible for the Administration of the CMHO. As mentioned, many staff responsible for operating CMHOs have primarily clinical backgrounds. They need specific training in financial and personnel management, marketing, program planning, budgeting, negotiating, and other generic management skills.

Budget Wisely for Present, as Well as Future, Corporate Needs. In the budgeting process, provisions must be made for depreciation of facilities. Reserves must be established for construction of new facilities, for new or expanded services, or for renovation of existing facilities. Adequate funds must be allocated for clinical and administrative staff training. A reserve should be developed for future paybacks in the event that a third-party funding source determines audit exceptions and requires reimbursement. Sufficient funds should be available for exploring and developing new ventures, for paying consultants required to determine financial feasibility of a new venture, to assist in obtaining a certificate of need for hospital beds, to assist in corporate reconfiguration, or to assist in improving management practices. The budgeting process must carefully examine how competitive the CMHO is when compared to other major health care providers in the local community and how competitive the CMHO is when recruiting for key positions at the state, regional, or national levels. The ability to attract and retain talented, well-qualified staff is essential if the long-term mission of the corporation is to be achieved. Each service department should be examined as a separate cost center and an evaluation made of its revenues and expenses. On its own, does the department (e.g., mental health adult outpatient services or substance abuse adolescent residential services) break-even financially, make a "profit," or lose money? If it loses money, what are the sources of funding that plug the deficit? Can the service department close the gap from deficit to break-even over a period of several years? If not, is the corporation willing to continue shifting funds to the service department to eliminate the deficit? Should the service be restructured to bring in more fee income? Should it be eliminated or merged with another service? These questions, and others, help the CMHO management team in the strategic budget planning required to keep the corporation out of financial difficulty and on the path of sound business practices.

Implement Effective Quality Assurance and Risk Management Programs. Although all CMHOs plan to provide high-quality services, many have not budgeted adequately nor allocated sufficient staff time to implement the quality assurance mechanisms necessary to evaluate and monitor services and to plan for the procedural and policy modifications necessary to continually improve service delivery. Specific staff time and CMHO resources must be dedicated to this important task, and frequently consultative assistance is necessary to design the quality control system. It is an ongoing process requiring numerous planning sessions and committee meetings. The standards of the Joint Commission on Accreditation of Healthcare Organizations can be extremely helpful in initiating and evaluating, over time, the CMHO's quality assurance activities. If the CMHO should elect to forego JCAHO accreditation, consultants familiar with the JCAHO accreditation process can still be of great help in developing and implementing an effective quality assurance plan. Other guidelines, of course, may be available from the state mental health/substance abuse authority, from the Commission on Accreditation of Rehabilitation Facilities, or other groups. (As an aside, many CMHOs consider JCAHO accreditation to be extremely valuable from the standpoint of increasing third-party reimbursement and quality of services, and they feel that accreditation will be increasingly important in the future.)

Risk management is of major importance in a CMHO's total quality assurance program. In addition to the need for an emphasis upon risk management from the standpoint of an ethical obligation to clients and staff, an effective risk management program is essential in our present litigious society. There is an ever-increasing number of professional liability lawsuits against CMHOs; obtaining and retaining adequate, affordable insurance will likely become a significant problem in the future. A well-established risk management program can assist in reducing the number of incidents that may give rise to a lawsuit, as well as better protect the health and safety of clients and staff. Risk management consultants are available in most larger communities. They can be of much assistance in reviewing and evaluating the risk management program operated by a CMHO and can provide specific recommendations for improvement in the risk management program.

Develop a Successful Marketing Program. When competing with other established health care providers (in contrast to providing services in programs that are primarily subsidized by the government), a CMHO must determine the nature and extent of marketing efforts necessary to attract the clientele required to fund the program. If the CMHO has been providing services to a medically indigent population and decides to diversify its funding base by establishing services that will be used by people who can pay full fee, then a marketing plan that has been well thought out must be developed to reach those people and let them know of the availability and desirability of the CMHO's services. Again, marketing skills must be learned by key management staff and funds set aside for necessary expert consultation and for the cost of marketing materials, purchase of advertising, and salary of CMHO staff involved in the various aspects of the marketing effort.

Develop an Active Foundation or Development Committee That Searches for the Philanthropic Dollar, Especially for the Purpose of Corporate Capital Needs. The development of a planned, organized approach to philanthrophy will have a long-term pay-off. Several years will be required to develop the ability of community volunteer board members to become successfully involved in a planned giving program. However, the additional funds obtained for services and facilities make possible growth that might not otherwise occur, as well as enhance the quality of services provided by the CMHO.

Consider Joint Ventures with Other Nonprofit or For-Profit Corporations. This is still a fairly new area for CMHOs but one that should be given serious consideration. Several CMHOs may jointly fund a new service to provide both additional community services and to operate as a profit center that can help fund CMHO indigent services that require subsidization. A

CMHO, for example, may enter into a joint venture with a for-profit hospital to build and operate a mental health or substance abuse facility. The hospital brings to the bargaining table access to capital for construction and the operational cash required until the new venture reaches the break-even point or becomes profitable. The CMHO brings to the table mental health and substance abuse treatment experience, reputation, community visibility, referrals, and understanding of the importance of continuity of care and case management, as well as some contribution of capital. Both organizations benefit.

Invest in Organizations That Can Assist in Continuing Strategic Planning Efforts, Technical Assistance, and Networking. Participation in such organizations should be considered to be a very cost-effective investment rather than a discretionary expense. Sharing ideas and experiences with other CMHOs at both the state and national level enables a CMHO to benefit from the hard-earned, expensive experience of others and reduces the learning curve when initiating new programs. These organizations include state CMHO associations, the National Council of Community Mental Health Centers, Mental Health Corporations of America, the Association of Mental Health Administrators (members may become qualified as certified mental health administrators), the American College of Mental Health Administration, the National Association of Private Psychiatric Hospitals, and other state and regional associations dealing, in varying degrees, with mental health treatment and administrative issues.

Understand the Advantages of Accreditation as it Relates to Improved Treatment and Increased Third-Party Reimbursement. Serious consideration should be given to budgeting the staff and financial resources necessary to obtain accreditation from such accrediting bodies as JCAHO. Although accreditation may not result in direct financial benefits in some states, in many states it can make the difference in whether or not insurance will pay for specific services provided by a CMHO. In addition to being cost-effective, preparation for accreditation serves as an excellent management review in areas of financial management, facilities review (fire and life safety issues), governance, training, quality assurance, risk management, and clinical records. Accreditation should not be perceived as an expense but rather viewed as a strategic investment.

Invest in Recruiting and Retaining Well-Trained, Experienced Clinical and Managerial Staff and Pay the Price Necessary to be Competitive with the For-Profit Sector. The not-for-profit CMHO must be able to compete effectively for the talent needed to assure effective management and continuation of high-quality services.

CONCLUSION

The private, nonprofit CMHO must understand the reality of the changes that are taking place in the industry and become willing and able to include in its vision of the future the creativity and the managerial flexibility required to become a viable and continuing part of health care delivery.

Morris L. Eaddy, PhD, is President and Chief Executive Officer of Lakeview Center, Inc. in Pensacola, Florida. He has worked in the field of community mental health for over 20 years and has served as President for The Florida Council for Community Mental Health, Mental Health Corporations of America, Mental Health Risk Retention Group, and as an officer of the Board of the National Council for Community Mental Health. In recent years, Lakeview Center has become actively involved in managed care contracts for mental health and substance abuse services. Dr. Eaddy may be contacted at Lakeview Center, 1221 W. Lakeview Avenue, Pensacola, FL 32501.

REFERENCES

Ambrose, D. M., & Lennox, L. (1988, Spring). Strategic market positions for mental health services. *Journal of Mental Health Administration, 15,* 5-9.

Boaz, J. T. (1988). *Delivering Mental Healthcare: A Guide for HMOs.* Chicago: Pluribus Press.

Del Pizzo, L., Byrd, J., Jr., & Smith, J. M. (1987, Winter). A strategic planning model for community mental health centers. *Administration in Mental Health,* pp. 91-101.

Ernst & Whinney (Accounting Firm). (1987). *Interim Progress Report for Mental Health Corporations of America, Inc..* Unpublished report prepared under contract with Mental Health Corporations of America, Inc., Tallahassee, FL.

Gapen, P. (1988, January 19). Reaching for the mental health market. *Health Week*, pp. 12-16.

Gaylin, S. (1985). The coming of the corporation and the marketing of psychiatry. *Hospital and Community Psychiatry, 36,* 154-159.

Kimmel, W. A. (1984). *The Role of the Private Sector in the Provision of Mental Health Services: An Exploratory Examination* (Office of State and Community Liaison, National Institute of Mental Health, DHHS, Alcohol, Drug Abuse and Mental Health Administration). Rockville, MD.

Kipp, M. F. (1984, Spring). *Lessons from the Private Sector.* Unpublished manuscript delivered as part of a series of symposia on The Financing of Mental Health Services.

Kipp, M. F. (1987, Spring). New directions for community mental health centers. *Journal of Mental Health Administration, 14,* 26-31.

Lee, F. C., & Schwartz, G. (1984, October). Paying for mental health care in the private sector. *Business and Health*, pp. 12-16.

National Institute of Mental Health. (1988, November 10). *Statistics.* DHHS, Alcohol, Drug Abuse, and Mental Health, Rockville, MD.

Neeley, J., & Ray, C. G. (1986a). *The Financial Marketing Management of Psychiatric Services: Strategic and Tactical Planning Aspects.* Proceedings for the Sixth Annual Symposium on Health Services Marketing and Academy for Health Services Marketing, Atlanta, GA.

Neeley, J, & Ray, C. G. (1986b). *Preparing for the Outcome-Oriented, Payor-Driven Marketplace.* Unpublished presentation at membership meeting of Mental Health Corporation of America, Inc., Houston, TX.

Perry, R. (1987, Spring). Survival is not enough--The case for profit. *Journal of Mental Health Administration, 14,* 37-39.

Rogers, P. (1986). *Trends and Innovations in Mental Health.* Arlington, VA: Capital Publications.

Schlesinger, M. (1985, January/February). The rise of proprietary health care. *Business and Health*, pp. 7-12.

Shea, J. G. (1986). *Competition in Mental Health: Opportunity or Threat?* Round-table discussion sponsored by E. R. Squibb and Sons. Published in *National Council News*, September, 1986.

Tsai, S. P., Reedy, S. M., & Bernacki, E. J. (1987, April). The effects of redesigning mental health benefits. *Business and Health*, pp. 26-28.

Wenzel, L. (1988, February). Mental health options under HMOs. *Business and Health*, pp. 30-33.

The Dual-
Disorder Client:
Mental Disorder and
Substance Use

Hilary Ryglewicz and Bert Pepper

One of the fascinating things about working in community mental health is the way in which new needs make themselves known. In general, new needs and new populations emerge as failures - in agencies' ability to provide effective treatment and in clients' ability to respond as expected.

Those who work on the front lines of public services encounter a great variety of clients, needs, and problems. These include people in psychotic episodes resulting from major mental illness; people in acute, suicidal depressions resulting from a life crisis; people with various combinations of emotional and interpersonal problems; people with medical and/or legal components to their difficulties; children and families in some form of emergency or crisis; and people who have abused alcohol and/or other drugs.

In general, the symptoms are expected to suggest the diagnosis; symptoms and diagnosis together determine the kinds of treatment and the level of care. Thus a person in an acute psychotic episode or with the symptom of suicidal and homicidal ideation goes into the psychiatric hospital - psychiatric treatment at the highest or most intensive level of care. The child and family presenting an emotional and behavioral crisis - provided there is no life-threatening behavior - are off to the outpatient clinic or child guidance agency. The alcohol abuser is placed on a detox unit - if he or she will stay - or engaged in alcohol outpatient treatment services, depending on the level of care that is currently required. The heroin addict is set up for methadone treatment. And so on.

Without these obvious, automatic associations of symptoms, diagnosis, and treatment services, emergency and crisis staff would be more hard-pressed than they are, if that were possible. If every case required us to sit down and ruminate about what would possibly be of help - to actually design services from scratch - the situation would be worthy of a Monty Python skit.

Yet, why does the description given here of staff plugging patients into services like happy switchboard operators sound overly rosy? Because we are grappling today with yet another new population, another new constellation of needs. The way new populations and their needs emerge is through treatment failure and, at the worst, system breakdown. Only when we have accumulated a number of such individual experiences of treatment and system failure do we begin to generalize and to seek adaptations in both treatment planning and system redesign.

THE NEW YOUNG
ADULT CLIENT POPULATION

During the decade of the 1980s the mental health service delivery system began to address the new phenomenon of the postdeinstitutionalization generation of people with severe, on-going mental disorders - the age group of 18 to 35 or 40 who were the first "chronic" or long-term clients to be served primarily in community outpatient care, often interspersed with "revolving door" hospital episodes.

This new generation were noted (Bachrach, 1982; Pepper, Kirshner, & Ryglewicz, 1981; Schwartz & Goldfinger, 1981; Sheets, Prevost, & Reihman, 1982) to show new constellations of symptoms and treatment needs in contrast to older patients who had spent much of their lives in institutional care. New and troubling concerns about these young men and women included their (a) resistance to becoming engaged in treatment; (b) frequent difficulty in diagnosis; (c) resistance toward or rejection of both specific treatment programs and the mental health system as a whole; (d) inappropriate use (overuse, underuse, misuse) of services; (e) high incidence of suicidal ideation, gestures, and attempts; (f) high incidence of volatile behavior and clashes with the law, as well as both family and social violence; (g) geographic restlessness and mobility; (h) high incidence of pregnancy and parenthood; and, not least (i) high incidence of use and abuse of alcohol and other drugs (Pepper & Ryglewicz, 1982).

74

This new generation of young adults was the first since the great convulsion of deinstitutionalization to grow into adulthood with serious mental disorders. Like their healthier age mates, they have been profoundly affected by the conditions of contemporary community life. Among these conditions, the most dangerous for the vulnerable person has been the widespread availability and casual use of alcohol and other drugs. Our present concern with "dual diagnosis" or "dual disorder" is in large part an outgrowth of the past decade's concern with today's population of young adults with ongoing mental disorders. There is substantial overlap between this larger group of clients in the age group 18 to 35 or 40 and the people we call "dual-disorder" clients. In many settings not only a sizable number but the *majority* of young adult psychiatric clients are reported to have problems with substance use.

DEINSTITUTIONALIZATION
AND THE DRUG-RIDDEN SOCIETY

If people with serious, ongoing mental disorders were still treated with long-term institutional care during much of their lives, they might be relatively insulated, as in the past, from the constant enticement to use drugs and alcohol, unless, of course, they obtained these substances from the staff or from people going out on pass. On the other hand, if alcohol and other drugs were not so ubiquitous in the society at this time, the hazards of community life for a psychiatrically vulnerable person would be greatly reduced.

Thirty years ago, institutional care was still the norm, *and*, although alcohol was widely used both during and after the failure of Prohibition, the use of other drugs was something known only on the fringes of society - among criminals and certain subgroups such as jazz musicians. It is not surprising, then, that "the mentally ill," "alcoholics," and "addicts" were seen as distinct populations with little, if any, overlap.

Today, young people with mental/emotional disorders are out in the community, *and* the community is awash with mind- and mood-altering drugs, of which alcohol is only the most publicly advertised. And today, we have substantial overlap between the population of people who use or abuse alcohol or street drugs and the population who suffer from serious, ongoing psychiatric problems.

75

It is important to recognize this dual-disorder population - in all its subgroups - as part of a much more far-reaching phenomenon in our society. Since the various revolutionary changes of the 1960s, it has been common for young people, as well as for many of the 1960s generation who have since become parents, to make routine "recreational" use of various kinds of drugs.

Alcohol is pushed constantly on TV, in the pages of magazines, on billboards, and in common parlance as the constant enabler of "a good time." Marijuana and then cocaine have come into widespread use as well. This affects not only marginal, minority, or disadvantaged populations, but a large proportion of the more privileged middle and upper socioeconomic classes. A range of other drugs (e.g., amphetamines, barbiturates, hallucinogens, "designer" drugs and other more imaginative concoctions) have also become more widely used, if less so than the big three: alcohol, marijuana, and cocaine. And it has become the norm for adolescents and young adults who use such substances to be polydrug users. That is, the populations of "alcoholics" and "drug addicts," which, like substance abusers and mentally ill people, used to be two distinct populations, are no longer separate groups. Younger people who drink are more than likely to use street drugs as well - and in many cases not merely one drug "of choice" but a variety, according to the moment and the mood.

The implications for community mental health agencies of this ever-spreading use and abuse of drugs are profound. Instead of working with distinct populations of "mentally ill" *or* substance-abusing people, each with a well-established protocol for treatment, we are trying to address ourselves to a mixed population with various symptom profiles and with multiple causative factors. In their interplay, these factors complicate assessment and treatment to a point where we have no recourse but change and adaptation in our treatment systems.

WHO IS THE DUAL-DISORDER CLIENT? FOUR SUBGROUPS

We use the term *dual-disorder* rather than *dually diagnosed*, *MICA* (Mentally Ill Chemical Abuser), *SAMI* (Substance Abusing Mentally Ill), and so on, and the term substance *use* or *use/abuse*, in order to stress a broad conception of this client population. In thinking about this population, we need to think in terms of at least four subgroups:

1. People with *major mental illness* involving intermittent psychotic episodes even without the use of alcohol and drugs, and more frequent and severe episodes when these substances are used. For this group, even minimal *use* further jeopardizes their mental/emotional stability.
2. People with *other psychiatric disorders such as severe personality disorder*, who suffer psychotic episodes *only* under the influence of alcohol and drug use. For this group, too, substance *use* at any level is a hazard, and there is a high potential for misdiagnosis.
3. People whose persistent alcohol and/or drug use/abuse/dependence/addiction (and sometimes other factors) may lead to and reinforce persistent *personality immaturity and dysfunction*. For this group, it is important to explore the relationship between the substance use and other patterns and skill deficits, as well as the level of the use or abuse itself.
4. People whose most obvious problem is alcohol and/or other substance use, but the use or withdrawal from use uncovers problematic symptoms and behavior. For this group, too, it is important to explore the circumstances, function, and consequences of the use and whether the person is substance-dependent or potentially able to exercise controls.

The first two of these groups are commonly referred to as *MICA* and are likely to be found in psychiatric treatment programs, including hospitals and crisis centers. People in the third and fourth groups may more commonly surface in substance abuse treatment programs, to which they may or may not be able to respond. Both the third and fourth groups may emerge - or go unnoticed - in mental health outpatient clinics. For any of these four subgroups of clients, it is vital to understand the interplay of mental/emotional disorder, personality immaturity and dysfunction, and substance use or abuse at any level.

MENTAL DISORDER AND SUBSTANCE USE: THE DEADLY INTERPLAY

The special hazards of alcohol and drug use for people with serious, persistent mental/emotional disorders are very well known to those who work on the front lines as caregivers. That includes, of course, parents and other family members as well as workers in treatment programs.

Briefly put: *Alcohol and drug use places an additional and often overwhelming stress on an already shaky and stress-vulnerable system.* That "system" may be understood as the brain, the body, the self, the ego, the person as a whole, and his or her relationships with others. Whatever the particular system or subsystem that is overstressed, the substance use is appropriately called "abuse" when it upsets an already tenuously held balance. For some people, the upsetting of that essential balance means another trip to the emergency room or another stay in the psychiatric hospital. For others, the consequence may be the loss of a job, quarrels with family members or a girlfriend, or a period of depression shown by staying home, not wanting to get out of bed, and so on.

When the substance use is clearly identified as *abuse* - as in the case of the usual *MICA* client or the person who comes to attention within the substance abuse system, it is not too difficult to see the effects of the alcohol or street drugs - in part because we are looking for them. These are clients who are clearly *abusing* the substance; that is, they are drinking or drugging enough so that people see their use as *too much* and see the effects of the substance in the form of symptoms. The connection is made, sometimes even by the person himself or herself, between the substance use and its effects and consequences.

Even though the connection is made, however, the dual-problem or dual-diagnosis client is often neglected or underserved by the treatment system. Typically, this client is the dual-problem victim of a single-problem program and receives appropriate attention to one but not both of his or her problems - the psychiatric disorder *or* the substance abuse.

For the person with a mental or personality disorder who merely *uses* alcohol and/or street drugs, the connection between substance use and symptoms usually is not so obvious, except to family or very close friends or staff who have lived through a number of episodes of fallout produced by so-called mild to moderate use. A parent says "My daughter can't pick up even one drink; she's not an alcoholic, but she's manic depressive, and she goes right out of control and back into the hospital." A young man says, "I know I shouldn't drink or smoke pot, because I get confused. But then, sometimes I think I can."

These are people who are *exquisitely sensitive* or *substance-vulnerable*. Their alcohol or drug use is often described as *not that much,* and they often have not been identified as needing any particular attention to their substance use. If the use has been noticed at all, it has been brushed aside as unimportant, or sympathized with as an attempt to be like everybody else. The observation that *even minimal substance use pushes the person "over the line" into thought disorder, mood disorder, unstable or aggressive behavior, or even psychosis* may not have been made.

In either the case of clear, overt substance *abuse* or minimal-to-moderate *use,* the person with a mental/emotional disorder may be at special risk of alcohol and drug effects. This special vulnerability may have any of three aspects:

1. *Chemical:* Just as some people are particularly sensitive to the effects of prescribed medications, the dual-disorder client may have a sensitivity to alcohol and street drugs that has to do with his or her *body chemistry* and particularly with direct effects upon the *brain.*

    Some people's brains appear especially vulnerable: that is, the immature, still-developing brain of a very young person; the aging brain of an older person; the brain that is impaired or compromised by learning disability or by schizophrenia; or the brain already damaged by substance use. For any of these reasons, a person's brain may be highly vulnerable to the disorganizing effects of substance use.

2. *Psychological:* A person with a mental/emotional/personality disorder has, by definition, some impairment of *ego functions* involving one or more of the capacities for judgment, reality testing, impulse control, affect modulation, memory, mastery, competence, and so forth.

    At the same time, we know very well that the characteristic impairments of the person who is under the influence of, say, alcohol, lie in precisely these areas. We know, too, that marijuana in high doses can produce hallucinations and paranoia; that psychedelic drugs distort perception, impair reality testing and judgment, and can produce both anxiety and hallucinations; that stimulants such as cocaine can produce anxiety, extremes of affect (euphoria, suicidal depression), and psychotic episodes; and so on.

    In other words, the more we as mental health professionals learn and reflect on the actual *specific* effects of alcohol and various street drugs, the more obvious it is that the "double trouble" of the dual-disorder client is very real, in psychological as well as chemical terms.

3. *Social*: Finally, the person with a mental/emotional disorder is vulnerable, not only chemically and psychologically, but also socially. The person's relationships and life situation may be only tenuously maintained: the job is one he or she has not had very long, so that he or she cannot afford to stay out late at night and come in foggy in the morning; the room is one in a series, with yet another landlady who is not pleased with any kind of erratic behavior; and/or the family or friend or lover already has lived through too many crises related to substance use.

This is a broader, more pervasive kind of vulnerability, but it is very real. Those people who have used up too much of their "social margin" through episodes of a psychiatric illness may pay an extra-heavy price for getting into trouble with alcohol and drugs.

These three kinds of vulnerability make it clear why a treatment system must concern itself with the dual-disorder client and must look beyond the boundaries of traditional methods and conceptions of its mission. And they also make clear why such clients so often emerge as treatment failures on one side of the service network or the other - in psychiatric *or* substance abuse treatment programs.

But, recalling that treatment failures are most fruitfully viewed as signals of unmet needs, this "failure" - often seen in and felt by clients and often also felt keenly by staff - must also be looked at from another perspective. It is also a "system failure" that reinforces the lack of a perceived connection between substance use or abuse and the persistence or worsening of psychiatric symptoms.

THE SINGLE-PROBLEM
TREATMENT SYSTEM

Failure of the treatment system to respond adequately to the needs of dual-disorder clients has three aspects: (a) limitations within the mental health system, (b) limitations within the substance abuse system, and (c) lack of integration between the two systems.

*THE MENTAL HEALTH TREATMENT
SYSTEM AND SUBSTANCE USE*

Until recently, mental health staff typically have been inattentive to problems of substance use and abuse. The usual limits of assessment have been expressed by the question: "Does the client drink or use drugs 'enough' to be sent to the alcohol/substance abuse system for treatment, or is his or her drinking or drugging not that much - that is, not more than what we now regard as expectable in our society?" Put more simply, the test sometimes may even be "Does the client drink more than his doctor, or smoke marijuana more than her mental health worker?"

The sources of this attitude are very clear:

1. *Alcohol and drug use, dependence and addiction, including its nature, frequency, general and specific effects, assessment, and treatment, has not been part of the training of most mental health staff.* Those who do have such knowledge generally have gained it informally, certainly not as a formal part of their repertoire for helping clients. The fact that some mental health staff *have* informed themselves and learned to work effectively in these areas is a tribute to their commitment and resourcefulness in their work, but it has not been a reliable expectation within mental health treatment programs. Consequently, the implications of substance *use* as well as abuse are easily overlooked, especially for the substance-vulnerable client.

2. *Formal assessment of substance use and abuse is also often overlooked in mental health treatment programs.* Workers who are unfamiliar with this area of inquiry are not likely to venture into it, nor to question the client thoroughly enough and with enough awareness of denial and downplaying of their use or abuse. None of us like to show our ignorance, especially if we do not know what we should or can do with the answers to our questions.

3. *If a mental health client is evaluated as having a mild to moderate substance use problem, the use is likely to be viewed as "self-medicating," and the treatment plan is likely to focus on addressing the psychiatric problems first.* The assumption is likely to be that the person drinks *because*

81

of his or her mental/emotional disturbance and that relief of the unmanageable emotions will automatically result in the disappearance of problematic substance use, especially if the use is viewed as "not that much."

4. *If a mental health client is evaluated as having a severe problem of substance abuse, the treatment plan is likely to be referral to a substance abuse treatment program, if that program will accept the client.* The rationale here is that the mental health program is not equipped to deal with the problem (usually true) or that it has no responsibility to treat the dual-disorder client (false).

5. *If it is clear that the client needs both psychiatric and substance abuse treatment, the usual question is: What should we do first?* That is, since concurrent, coordinated treatment is not typically available in most settings, the only choice is to offer one and then the other sequentially. Unfortunately, this does not work because the client does not "get over" either disorder, especially when each is treated in isolation from the other.

6. *The mental health treatment program typically has not been either motivated or equipped to offer education about substance use and its effects.* Where at least some of the "treatment" needed is educational or didactic in its nature, mental health staff have not been accustomed to education as a treatment modality, nor have they had the necessary knowledge or sense of expertise in this area.

7. *The mental health treatment program, unlike a substance abuse treatment program, is not necessarily committed to a goal of abstinence, but more likely to a goal of "not too much" substance use for its clients.* Accordingly, staff of the program may not attempt to engage clients in working toward abstinence, but rather may view "mild" or "moderate" drinking and drug use as normal: as one of the person's few sources of pleasure and as necessary to the person's efforts to socialize.

Historically, and in many cases extending into the present, these have been the limitations that have caused the substance-using or abusing client to be poorly served within the mental health treatment system. Fortunately, these attitudes and other limitations are changing, as will be outlined below.

THE SUBSTANCE ABUSE TREATMENT SYSTEM AND THE PERSON WITH A MENTAL/EMOTIONAL DISORDER

If the mental health treatment system often has failed the dual-disorder client, the situation has not been any better in the substance abuse treatment system. Whether or not the treating agency is part of an overarching mental health delivery system that includes substance abuse treatment, there are generally problems in delivering customary modes of treatment to a person who also has a serious psychiatric disorder, and it is difficult for such programs to adapt their approaches to the needs of such a client, even if the need for some modification is recognized.

The usual limitations of the substance abuse treatment program in serving dual-disorder clients parallel those of the mental health system:

1. *The mental disorders, including major mental illness and severe personality disorder, have not been part of the training of most substance abuse staff.* Indeed, the usual perspective of the substance abuse treatment program, with its essential focus upon the *primary* importance of the substance disorder, tends to militate against a concern with differential diagnosis in the psychiatric sense.
2. *Consequently, it is easy for staff to misinterpret certain responses of dual-disorder clients as "resistance" or "denial."* When the vulnerabilities involved in specific mental illnesses are unfamiliar, it is natural to feel that the person is not cooperating with treatment. It is also natural to press issues and confront behaviors more insistently than may be appropriate for a given client.
3. *Psychiatric evaluation and differential diagnosis is not typically a formal part of assessment in a substance abuse program.* Rather, psychiatric evaluation may be utilized for those clients who are already perceived as "treatment resistant" or "treatment failures." This may result in client's being excluded by the program or referred to a psychiatric treatment program.
4. *If the client is troubled with severe anxiety or depression, these symptoms are likely to be interpreted as secondary to the substance abuse and the process of achieving abstinence, or as attempts to manipulate the situation by requesting medication.* The need to overcome a tendency to

seek chemical relief from painful emotions is necessarily a basic tenet of the substance abuse program.

5. *If a substance abuse client is identified as having a serious mental/emotional disorder that interferes with his or her response to treatment, the outcome is likely to be referral to another (psychiatric) program rather than adaptation of the substance abuse treatment protocol.* The rationale is that the program is designed for the majority and is not equipped to adapt to the needs of mentally ill people. Or, if the mental disorder is not perceived as so severe as to preclude substance abuse treatment on the usual models, the demands of the program are likely to be maintained; the client may withdraw, bolt, or wander from treatment.

6. *The substance abuse treatment program is specifically directed to the goal of abstinence; it is not oriented to working over time with a pre-abstinent and unmotivated client who is not ready to undertake this goal.* If it is clear that the client needs both substance abuse and psychiatric treatment, the question "What should we do first?" would normally be answered "Achieve abstinence." However, if the client is not yet motivated for abstinence, the program may require the development of motivation as a prerequisite for program participation. Motivation for abstinence can be very difficult to develop for the client with a mental disorder, who may have trouble with *all* aspects of motivation, reality testing, judgment, and goal-directed effort. In fact, it can require patient effort over a period of years.

7. *The substance abuse treatment program, unlike a psychiatric treatment program, is not necessarily committed to the principles of outreach, individualized treatment, and maintaining the person in treatment through any necessary adaptations.* Rather than viewing the client as someone who must be kept in treatment if at all possible, the substance abuse treatment program is likely to place a greater weight upon the need to maintain its integrity as a goal-directed group milieu and on the need of the individual to comply with its principles and purposes. This priority is appropriate in terms of the need of the program to place the strongest possible structure in opposition to the power of alcohol/drug dependence and addiction. But, for the dual-disorder client who has not yet learned to recognize the value and necessity of absti-

come familiar with the entire range of psychiatric disorders and their symptoms.

Dual-Disorder Treatment as a Track in a Substance Abuse Program. This model may become more familiar as substance abuse staff become sensitized to the dual-disorder client and his or her psychiatric problems and dysfunctional responses to the program. As in mental health, the dual-disorder client often emerges as a "treatment failure" or "revolving door client" - the revolving door being, in this case, the one between the two treatment systems. Dual-disorder clients with severe substance abuse problems certainly could be well-served in a special track of substance abuse treatment. Disadvantages of this approach might be:

1. Difficulty in modifying treatment approaches sufficiently to serve clients' needs concerning possible cognitive impairments, vulnerability to overstimulation, or poor affective modulation.
2. Reluctance to prescribe even nonaddictive psychotropic medications that are needed for clients' psychiatric symptoms may be important in maintaining abstinence.
3. Difficulty in setting limits for the pre-abstinent and unmotivated client - abstinence being a clear-cut goal of the program - without jeopardizing the continuity of psychiatric treatment.
4. Difficulty in maintaining a less confrontational, slower-moving track for such clients in the midst of a larger population that, apart from the problem of addiction, is commonly more socially functional, and in the context of a program with a strong commitment to abstinence.
5. Inadequate numbers for a special track, because more dual-disorder clients are likely to emerge in the psychiatric treatment program, where they are not referred or maintained because of substance abuse, but because of their symptoms of mental/emotional disorder.

The Dual-Disorder (MICA) Program as a Special Unit. In theory, the creation of a special unit with its own integrated program design and staff representing both psychiatric and substance abuse disciplines has much to recommend it. Such a program generally serves as a model and is specially funded, with access to enriched resources and more intensive staffing. However, like any model or demonstration project, such a program is often at risk in its continued survival in terms of both funding and numbers of clients served, as well as in the continuation of its "special" resources and staffing. Often its applicability to another setting is in question, or it is not replicable because of the special resources required. Even without such considerations, a dual-disorder track within a program seems more readily able to draw upon resources of the main program and is readily accessed by clients without unnecessary labeling. A key to working with dual-disorder clients is accomplishing engagement in a manner that permits the *client* to come to the conclusion that he or she has a problem with substance use.

TREATMENT MODALITIES
FOR THE DUAL-DISORDER CLIENT

For the long-term mental health client, as well as for the person in substance abuse treatment, a multi-modal approach is needed, including:

1. *Education/psychoeducation concerning alcohol/drug use and its effects*, with special attention to what substance use or abuse means for the dual-disorder client.
2. *Development of alternative coping skills* to compensate for personality immaturity and replace substance use as a dysfunctional coping effort. Stress management, problem-solving, communication, and other personal and interpersonal skills are relevant.
3. *Medication education, monitoring, and self-monitoring*, including education about medication effects, differences between prescribed medication use and alcohol or street drug use, and so on.
4. *Vocational/educational/social remediation and support* to address deficits in functioning in these areas that have resulted from each or both disorder(s). These supports may take the form of new initiatives in transitional programs (Ryglewicz, 1987; Unger, 1987) as well as more traditional approaches.
5. *Physical activity, education, and support* including exercise, nutrition, working with other forms of addiction (e.g., eating disorders, cigarette smoking, caffeine), and so on.

EDUCATION AND PSYCHOEDUCATION
IN DUAL-DISORDER TREATMENT

In all of these areas, an educational/psychoeducational approach has important advantages. Psychoeducation as a modality, which is receiving increasing attention as a beneficial and nonstigmatizing way of conveying much of the content of "treatment" (Hendrickson, 1989; Ryglewicz, 1989a) is particularly valuable in working with dual-disorder clients as well as families (Ryglewicz, 1989b; Sciacca, 1989). In fact, we advocate an educational approach as the core of the program, especially for the unmotivated or pre-abstinent client.

The rationale for this lies in the nonstigmatizing and non-pejorative quality of an educational approach, as well as the very real need to convey a basic knowledge base about alcohol and drug use and its effects; vulnerability to small amounts of use, medications and their differences from street drugs, and so on.

ATTENTION TO NEUROPSYCHOLOGICAL
DEFICITS OF DUAL-DISORDER CLIENTS

Reports of deficits in neuropsychological functioning among people with mental disorders or past or current substance use (Grant et al., 1979; Zacker, Pepper, & Kirshner, 1989) suggest a need for further exploration of this area and for programming that is tailored to address and modify such deficits. An innovative program based at the Rockland County Department of Mental Health (Project SHIFT, operated by The Information Exchange under a grant from New York State's Integrated Task Force for dual-disorder youth) has utilized teaching modules and computer technology to provide individually designed targeting of learning and coping skills for young adults with various diagnoses. However, this kind of work is appropriate only when the person has achieved a period of abstinence, because substance use precludes both accurate evaluation and effective learning in this area.

A RANGE OF INTERVENTIONS
FOR THE DUAL-DISORDER CLIENT

Above all, it is desirable as a program matures to offer a range of groups and other options to address the needs of clients at various levels of use and abuse and various stages of motivation and efforts toward abstinence. The particular content, format, and number of such groups may vary according to a given agency's resources and client needs. The essence of such a program is the provision of a range of interventions addressing not only the development of motivation for abstinence, but also the development of skills to support abstinence and protect against relapse.

Like other serious, ongoing major mental/emotional disorders, substance abuse and substance dependence are never "over"; the achievement of sobriety or abstinence is only the beginning of a long road. For most people this road is rocky and winding, and it must include a great deal of work on past deficits in skills and experience as well as the emotional process of "forgiving the past." In the beginning of alcohol/substance abuse treatment an enormous amount of energy is devoted to developing motivation and achieving the beginning of abstinence. As the road continues the work shifts to the maintenance of abstinence and the prevention of relapse. Only by developing new skills, habits, associations, ways of relating to oneself and other people does the substance-dependent or substance-abusing person become better able to walk on solid ground.

For people with dual disorders, the complications of major mental illness or entrenched personality disorder are sometimes overwhelming. For many clients both sobriety and stability are elusive goals or are only tenuously maintained. This is because it is so difficult to establish new personal or interpersonal skills, and the fluctuations of illness and life stress continue to limit or compromise achievement in these areas. It is vital for treatment staff to recognize these problems and commit themselves to maximum patience and maximum outreach with dual-disorder clients.

WORKING WITH SELF-HELP GROUPS

Helping clients to utilize self-help groups such as Alcoholics Anonymous (AA) and Narcotics Anonymous (NA) is a crucial component in dual-disorder treatment. The potential value of a strong supportive culture and the structure of a 12-step program is enormous. At the same time, it is crucial to offer special support to dual-disorder clients in their use of self-help groups.

Specifically, treatment staff may need to (a) help with transportation to AA/NA meetings, (b) help clients to identify meetings where their mental/emotional problems are accepted, (c) educate and support clients about their use of necessary psychotropic medications, (d) adapt the 12-step approach and other messages of AA/NA to include the dual aspects of their problems, and (e) help clients to form and maintain "double trouble" self-help groups if their needs are not met in local AA/NA meetings.

STAFF TRAINING NEEDS
FOR THE DUAL-DISORDER CLIENT

Clearly this provision of effective programs for the dual-disorder client requires intensive and extensive work in training staff in both mental health and substance abuse programs. Cross-trainings that present a sound knowledge base concerning substance use and its effects, substance abuse treatment principles, mental disorders and their symptoms and treatment, and so on, are sorely needed.

Particular emphasis must be placed upon (a) the interaction of psychiatric and substance use disorders; (b) the substance-vulnerable client who disorganizes with even minimal use; (c) strategies, techniques, and philosophies for developing motivation for abstinence; (d) ways of dealing with conflict between approaches and perspectives of the mental health and substance abuse treatment systems; and (e) guidelines for providing support without "enabling" for the pre-abstinent or unmotivated dual-disorder client.

EVALUATION AND TREATMENT:
AN ONGOING INTERPLAY

Above all, it is vital to insure that both mental health and substance abuse agencies develop protocols and tools to provide:

1. *Evaluation at the entry point* that includes a thorough assessment of substance use or abuse as well as a careful assessment of mental status and psychosocial functioning. Such evaluation may necessarily include gathering information from the social network, including family.
2. *Treatment planning* that includes attention and interventions concerning substance use as well as psychiatric symptoms and personal/social deficits, involving both treatment systems as needed and insofar as possible.
3. Ongoing evaluation and treatment planning and monitoring so that the initial decision about the location and plan

for treatment can be periodically reviewed and revised, based on experience with the client.

Treatment agencies today are struggling to overcome our long-practiced tendency to base treatment plans and referrals for dual-disorder clients upon "either/or" decisions made too close to the front door. The task is to achieve an integration of the perspectives and expertise of both psychiatric and substance abuse treatment systems, so that we can take a truly cooperative and coordinated approach to evaluation and treatment of the *MICA* or dual-disorder population.

Enhancing the sensitivity of mental health staff to problems of substance use and of substance abuse staff to psychiatrically based impairments can take us a long way down that road. The remaining work will be to develop a shared perspective, coherent strategy, and cooperative techniques for developing motivation for abstinence among "double trouble" clients.

Hilary Ryglewicz, ACSW, is currently Clinical Assistant to the Commissioner of Mental Health and Coordinator of Family/Consumer Services at the Rockland County New York Department of Mental Health. She is also Training/Publications Coordinator for The Information Exchange (TIE), Inc. and Contributing Editor of its quarterly bulletin, *TIE-LINES.* She is a nationally known trainer and consultant on dual-diagnosis treatment and programming. Ms. Ryglewicz may be contacted at Rockland County Department of Mental Health, Building F, Pomona, NY 10970.

Bert Pepper, MD, is Founder and Executive Director of The Information Exchange (TIE), Inc. and a former Commissioner of Mental Health in Rockland County, New York. He has served as president of the American Orthopsychiatric Association, as Director, Consultation Service of the American Psychiatric Association, as Clinical Professor of Psychiatry, New York University School of Medicine, and as Lecturer, Johns Hopkins University. He is a nationally known consultant and trainer on dual-diagnosis treatment and programming. Dr. Pepper can be contacted at The Information Exchange (TIE), Inc., 20 Squadron Boulevard, Suite 400, New City, NY 10956.

REFERENCES

CITED REFERENCES

Bachrach, L. L. (1982). Young adult chronic patients: An analytical review of the literature. *Hospital and Community Psychiatry, 33,* 189-197.

Grant, I., Reed, R., Adams, K., & Carlin, A. (1979). Neuropsychological function in young alcoholics and polydrug abusers. *Journal of Clinical Neuropsychology, 1,* 39-47.

Hendrickson, E. L. (1989, April). Taking a look at psychoeducation/a group for dual-disorder clients. *TIE-LINES, VI*(2), 3-5.

Pepper, B., Kirshner, M. C., & Ryglewicz, H. (1981). The young adult chronic patient: Overview of a population. *Hospital and Community Psychiatry, 32,* 463-469.

Pepper, B., & Ryglewicz, H. (1982, June). The uninstitutionalized generation: A new breed of psychiatric patient. In B. Pepper & H. Ryglewicz (Eds.), *The Young Adult Chronic Patient: New Directions for Mental Health Services* (Vol. 14). San Francisco: Jossey-Bass.

Ryglewicz, H. (1987, April). Teaching as treatment: A path out of patienthood. *TIE-LINES, IV*(II), 1-2.

Ryglewicz, H. (1989a, April). Psychoeducation: A wave of the present. *TIE-LINES, VI*(2), 1-2.

Ryglewicz, H. (1989b, July). Psychoeducational work with families: Theme and variations. *TIE-LINES, VI*(3), 1-3.

Schwartz, S., & Goldfinger, S. (1981). The new chronic patient: Clinical characteristics of an emerging subgroup. *Hospital and Community Psychiatry, 32,* 470-474.

Sciacca, K. (1989, July). MICAA-Non: Working with families, friends and advocates of mentally ill chemical abusers and addicted (MICAA). *TIE-LINES, VI*(3), 7-8.

Sheets, J. L., Prevost, J. A., & Reihman, J. (1982). Young adult chronic patients: Three hypothesized subgroups. *Hospital and Community Psychiatry, 33,* 197-203.

Unger, K. (1987, April). A university-based rehabilitation program. *TIE-LINES, IV*(II), 2-3.

Zacker, J., Pepper, B., & Kirshner, M. C. (1989). Neuropsychological characteristics of young adult chronic psychiatric patients: Preliminary observations. *Perceptual and Motor Skills, 68,* 391-399.

ADDITIONAL SOURCES

Books

Alterman, A. I. (Ed.). (1985). *Substance Abuse and Psychopathology*. New York: Plenum.

Daley, D. C., Moss, H., & Campbell, F. (1987). *Dual Disorders: Counseling Clients with Chemical Dependency and Mental Illness*. Center City, MN: Hazelden.

Donovan, D. M., & Marlatt, G. A. (Eds.). (1988). *Assessment of Addictive Behaviors*. New York: Guilford.

Evans, K., & Sullivan, J. M. (1990). *Dual Diagnosis: Counseling the Mentally Ill Substance Abuser*. New York: Guilford.

Gottheil, E., McLellan, A. T., & Druly, K. A. (1980). *Substance Abuse and Psychiatric Illness*. New York: Pergamon.

Meyer, R. E. (1986). *Psychopathology and Addictive Disorders*. New York: Guilford.

Articles

Ananth, J., Vandewater, S., Kamal, M., Brodsky, A., Gamal, R., & Miller, M. (1989, March). Missed diagnosis of substance abuse in psychiatric patients. *Hospital and Community Psychiatry, 40*(3).

Brown, V. B., Ridgely, M. S., Pepper, B., Shifren-Levine, I., & Ryglewicz, H. (1989, March). The dual crisis: Mental illness and substance abuse: Present and future directions. *American Psychologist, 44*, 565-569.

Caton, C. L. M., Gralnick, A., Bender, S., & Simon. R. (1989, October). Young chronic patients and substance abuse. *Hospital and Community Psychiatry, 40*, 1037-1040.

Cote, W. R., & Lisnow, F. (1985, March/April). The substance abuser in crisis: Evaluation and treatment. *The Counselor*.

Crowley, T. (1974, January). Drug and alcohol abuse among psychiatric admissions. *Archives of General Psychiatry, 30*.

Drake, R. E., McLaughlin, P., Pepper, B., & Minkoff, K. (1991). Dual diagnosis of major mental illness and substance disorder: An overview. In K. Minkoff & R. E. Drake (Eds.), *New Directions for Mental Health Services* (Vol. 50, pp. 3-9). San Francisco: Jossey-Bass.

Drake, R. E., & Wallach, M. A. (1989, October). Substance abuse among the chronic mentally ill. *Hospital and Community Psychiatry, 40,* 1041-1046.
Fariello, D., & Scheidt, S. (1989, October). Clinical case management of the dually diagnosed patient. *Hospital and Community Psychiatry, 40*(10).
Kanwischer, R. W., & Hundley, J. (1990, July). Screening for substance abuse in hospitalized psychiatric patients. *Hospital and Community Psychiatry, 41*(7).
Lehman, A. F., Myers, C. P., & Corty, E. (1989, October). *Hospital and Community Psychiatry, 40*(10).
Minkoff, K. (1989, October). An integrated treatment model for dual diagnosis of psychosis and addiction. *Hospital and Community Psychiatry, 40,* 1031-1036.
Osher, F. C., & Kofoed, L. L. (1989, October). Treatment of patients with psychiatric and psychoactive substance abuse disorders. *Hospital and Community Psychiatry, 40,* 1025-1030.
Regier, D. A., Farmer, M. E., Rae, D. P., Locke, B. Z., Keith, S. J., Judd, L. L., & Goodwin, F. K. (1990, November 21). Comorbidity of mental disorders with alcohol and other drug abuse: Results from the Epidemiologic Catchment Area (ECA) Study. *Journal of the American Medical Association, 264,* 2511-2518.
Ryglewicz, H. (1991, October). Psychoeducation for clients and families: A way in, out, and through in working with people with dual disorders. *Psychosocial Rehabilitation Journal, 15,* 79-89.
Safer, D. J. (1987, May). The young adult chronic patient and substance abuse. *Hospital and Community Psychiatry, 38,* 511-514.

RESOURCE MATERIALS

Mental Illness and Substance Abuse: The Dually Diagnosed Client. Rockville, MD: National Council of Community Mental Health Centers.
Ridgely, M. S., Goldman, H. H., & Talbott, J. A. *Chronically Mentally Ill Young Adults with Substance Abuse Problems: A Review of Relevant Literature and Creation of a Research Agenda.* Baltimore, MD: Mental Health Policy Studies, Department of Psychiatry, University of Maryland School of Medicine.

Ridgely, M. S., Osher, F. C., & Talbott, J. A. *Chronically Mentally Ill Young Adults with Substance Abuse Problems: Treatment and Training Issues*. Baltimore, MD: Mental Health Policy Studies, Department of Psychiatry, University of Maryland School of Medicine.

Developing
Comprehensive
Mental Health Services
in Local Jails and
Police Lockups

Gerald Landsberg

There is a growing and imperative need that community
mental health agencies establish extensive linkages with local
correctional facilities to develop comprehensive mental health
services systems for these institutions. Jails and police lockups
are serving increasing numbers of both the seriously and persist-
ently mentally ill populations in acute psychiatric distress:

> The rate of suicides in jails is nine times that of the gen-
> eral population. (Hayes, 1989, p. 16)

> Some 600,000 mentally ill individuals are among the
> 7,000,000 people incarcerated in our county and city
> operated jails every year. (National Coalition for Jail
> Reform, 1984, p. 1)

Yet, overall, these local jails and lockups have extremely limited
access to community based mental health services. Rather, jail-
mental health interaction is frequently one of avoidance, suspi-
cion, and mistrust, characterized by the comment: "It isn't
whether you win or lose, but where you place the blame . . . no
one wants to be responsible for the problem" (Chaiklin, 1986, p.
16).

In this chapter, the need for mental health services in jails will
be reviewed. Specifically, data on the high rate of suicides in jails
and the increasing pressures on jails from courts (via financial
liability awards) to address the issue will be presented. This will

be followed by information on the increasing numbers of chronically mentally ill that are being incarcerated and a discussion of the dilemma of jails (i.e., lack of appropriate personnel, the difficulty in transferring patients to psychiatric facilities) in adequately serving these populations. The development of mental health programs in jails will be discussed, followed by discussion of the need for an interagency conceptual agreement, a model of comprehensive jail mental health services, and strategies for funding.

THE NEED FOR MENTAL HEALTH SERVICES IN JAILS

Over the past two decades, the need to serve the mentally distressed and the chronically mentally ill in our jails and local correctional facilities is becoming more evident. There are two primary indicators of this need: suicides (and attempted suicides) and the increasing incarceration of the chronically mentally ill.

JAIL SUICIDES

Susan Charle (1981) dramatically described the issue of jail suicides as follows:

> On Nov. 29, 1980, a 16-year-old John Russell Hayden was imprisoned in the Hamilton County (Ohio) Juvenile Detention Center. A few hours after his arrest, Hayden tied a bedsheet to the bars of his cell and hanged himself. He had been arrested for truancy. . . .
> . . . at least 11 who killed themselves during a two week period from Nov. 29 to Dec. 13, 1980 in police lockups and jails from Worcester, Mass. to Spokane, Wash. And the 11 were only a few of the hundreds of inmates in jails and prisons who kill themselves every year. Suicide among prisoners is an acute and growing problem. (p. 1)

Suicide is the leading cause of death in the nation's jails and police lockups. Studies have shown rates of jail suicides of *three to nine times* the general population (Danto, 1973; Hayes, 1989; National Center on Institutions and Alternatives, 1981). In fact, it is the more recent comprehensive study (Hayes, 1989) that suggests the rate of jail suicides is nine times that of the general population (12.3 suicides per 100,000 for the general population versus 107 suicides per 100,000 inmate population; Hayes, 1989).

Heightening concern over suicide is not only this significant rate, but also the fact that increasing litigation associates with suicide and suicide attempts has grown markedly; courts are often finding in favor of the plaintiffs and awarding substantial liability payments. The impact of this liability issue is noted in the court decision described below:

> *Shepherd v. Dickson County Sheriff's Department*, U.S. District Court (Charlotte, Tenn. 1984). A federal court awarded survivors of a man arrested for public drunkenness $600,000 for the negligent death of the man. The court found that county deputies should have taken the arrestee to the hospital, as they were advised by a woman at the scene of the arrest that she saw the man swallow a bottle of pills.
>
> The deputies transported the prisoner to the jail instead, and placed him in the drunk tank, which he occupied alone. He died several hours later from a drug overdose. (*Detention Reporter*, 1986, p. 9)

This legal action, and concerns of jail personnel, have left administrators and staff greatly concerned about this issue.

JAILS AS PLACES OF CONFINEMENT FOR SERIOUSLY MENTALLY ILL

Studies show that the chronically mentally ill are increasingly being confined for periods of time at local correctional facilities. Results from these studies suggest that 2% to 8% of the jail population have psychotic disorders (Bogira, 1981; Bolton, 1976; Valdiserri, Carroll, & Hartl, 1986) and that as many as 24% have prior histories of psychiatric inpatient treatment (Callahan & Diamond, 1985; Chaiklin, 1986; Massachusetts Department of Mental Health, 1980; Steadman & Ribner, 1980; New York State Office of Mental Health (1991). The National Coalition for Jail Reform (1984) eloquently writes:

> The nation's 3,493 local jails are increasingly becoming the dumping grounds for the mentally ill people in our communities. By recent estimates, some 600,000 mentally ill individuals are among the 7,000,000 people incarcerated in our county and city operated jails every year.

Many of these people are chronically mentally ill. Their crimes are often less the result of criminal intent than an inability to function in their communities. Many are picked up for becoming unruly or acting out in the street, the bus station or the diner. They are charged with disturbing the peace, trespassing, and other minor crimes.

Most of these people are not a danger to the community. But they are troublesome--to their families and neighbors, to the agencies which attempt to serve them, to the businesses they frequent. They are troublesome to the criminal justice system and to the mental health system. . . .

With greater numbers of people in the community needing mental health care and fewer mental health services available, there are more mentally ill people acting out on the streets or facing crises and thus coming to the attention of the police. (p. 2)

Perhaps most dramatically, the case below illustrates this problem:

After 14 years in state mental health institutions, 58-year-old Helen was discharged back to her small-town community where she shared an apartment with her elderly sister. Within one year of her hospital discharge, she had been jailed seven times on such minor charges as disorderly conduct, trespassing and creating a public nuisance. According to the local sheriff, her sister was unable to control her, the mental hospital would not take her back and "there is no where else to put her." (Craig & Kissell, 1988, p. 1)

Commenting further on the "criminalizing mental disorder," Teplin (1984), based upon her National Institute of Mental Health funded study, comments:

In the present study, it was common practice for the police to obtain a signed complaint in situations where the person was thought by the police to require psychiatric hospitalization. The logic underlying this procedure was to ensure the ready availability of an alternative disposition (arrest) in the event that the hospital found the individual unacceptable for admission. The police officer's apparent ingenuity was clearly born out of necessity because hospitals have very specific criteria for admission . . . every police officer was aware of the rather stringent requirements for admission into the local psychiatric hospital. . . . Police knew that persons who were mentally retarded, alcoholic or defined by hospital staff to be "dangerous" were persona non grata at the hospital. . . . Thus, the criminal justice system may have become the "court of last resort" because, unlike other agencies, it has no requirements or restrictions for entry. (p. 800)

OBSTACLES IN SERVICES
TO THE MENTALLY ILL IN JAILS

Jails and jail staff are, in fact, ill equipped to serve the mentally disturbed and the chronically mentally ill. Historically, jails and police lockups were never *built* nor *staffed* to provide the sophisticated components of classification, treatment, and observation that are now expected of them.

GROWTH IN INMATE POPULATIONS

Exacerbating the problem of handling the mentally ill is the fact that the correctional system in the United States is bursting at the seams. "Over the past decade, the nation's prison population has almost doubled. In 1975, there were 240,593 in state and federal prisons, while in 1986 there were over 546,659. In June, 1984, there were 234,500 detainees in jails. . . . One in 500 Americans is currently behind bars. . . . Prison and jail construction have not kept pace with needs. The shortage of federal and state beds is over 113,999" (Atlas, 1989, p. 158).

The consequences of this lack of prison space are multiple: (a) nearly half the nation's inmates are convicted felons (as compared to pretrial and misdemeanor defendants); (b) jails, like prisons, have become places of growing violence; and (c) with prison and jail construction falling further behind, correctional facilities are getting older and older. Eighty-one percent of the jails operating in 1980 were built before 1969. Thus, the environmental factor often encourages suicidal or "acting out" behaviors (Atlas, 1989).

LACK OF APPROPRIATE PERSONNEL

Comparatively little research has focused on the availability of mental health services provided by jails, but an examination of key data on the availability of health care would strongly suggest that mental health care is not a high priority. For example, 62% of jails have no doctor available on a regularly scheduled basis and only 128 jails out of 3,493 are accredited by the American Medical Association for adequate health services (National Coalition for Jail Reform, 1984). Morrissey et al. (1984) suggest that "given the paucity of any human services in most jails, it is clear that most of the 157,000 inmates in these facilities on any given day do not have access to proper mental health care" (p. 236).

This lack of proper mental health care can possibly be attributed to several facts: (a) a very large percentage of our jails are small (i.e., 44% have fewer than 10 inmates) and, thus, lack mental health resources (National Coalition for Jail Reform, 1984); (b) "traditionally, given the rapid turnover of inmates and a mandate mainly for safe retention until criminal disposition, jail authorities and county fiscal officers have not defined mental health services as a jail responsibility" (Morrissey et al., 1984, p. 236); and (c) historically, inmates with severe psychiatric and behavioral problems were transferred to state mental hospitals that were used as primary providers; these are no longer available (Morrissey et al., 1984).

DIFFICULTY IN TRANSFERRING
PATIENTS TO PSYCHIATRIC FACILITIES

Compounding the growth of the overall jail population and the lack of appropriate personnel, jails are also confronted with limited ability to transfer inmates to psychiatric institutions. The factors that limit the ability to transfer include (a) the reduction in long-term psychiatric care beds in state hospitals, (b) the widespread reluctance of short-term psychiatric care facilities to accept jail or criminal justice clients, and (c) the imposition of stringent standards for involuntary commitments for psychiatric care. The fact that jail personnel are not independent agents and, thus, are not readily able to take action to transfer or release mentally ill inmates without actions by the court and/or district attorney's office also can complicate transfers.

THE GAPS BETWEEN
SYSTEMS: AN OVERVIEW

In examining the difficulty between mental health and jail systems, it is clear that:

- Communications between the two systems are inadequate.
- Formal agreements with respect to mutual obligations for the mentally ill offender are few.
- Mental health staff frequently are unaware of the criminal justice system's problems with the mentally ill offender as well as its overall role and responsibilities.
- Jail staffs frequently lack the skills to identify and manage mental health problems.
- The two systems frequently approach the problem from two differing philosophies - punishment versus treatment.

The lacks in coordination between the two systems have a substantial negative impact on both systems as well as on the mentally ill offender needing care (Chaiklin, 1986; Craig & Kissel, 1988; New York State Office of Mental Health, 1991).

LACK OF INTERAGENCY CONCEPTUAL
AGREEMENTS: A FUNDAMENTAL FLAW

Evidence indicates that *a*, if not *the*, primary difficulty in establishing mental health-jail program services is the frequent lack of a common agreement between the mental health and the correctional agency on the questions: "What is the problem?" "Who should be serviced?" "What services should be provided?" From the observations below, a perspective on this issue can be offered:

Brodsky (1987) notes:

A ... dilemma arises in the case of violent and disordered persons: neither agency wants such persons in its care. The hospital is frightened by the violence and does not have secure facilities. The jail is frightened by the severity of the psycho-pathology and does not have the staff or facilities appropriate to deal with psychotic prisoners. It is not unusual for reciprocal blame and ill-will to be generated by the agency interactions about these prisoners. . . . Different expectations and objectives for the collaboration produce poor communication and resentment. (p. 3)

Chaiklin (1986) quoted the Maryland Criminal Justice Coordinating Council, 1984, report on mentally ill offenders as follows:

. . . a major definitional problem surrounds the issue of mentally ill offenders. No agency in the state has developed a comprehensive definition of the chronically mentally ill that is applicable to the mentally ill offender population. Although the Mental Hygiene Administration (MHA) and the Division of Correction (DOC), among other agencies, have developed their own operation definitions, a uniform definition has not been developed. For example, for planning purposes, the Division of Correction considers an inmate to be mentally ill if they have had a prior hospitalization for mental illness; MHA defines chronically mental ill as being diagnosed as a schizophrenic, major affective, organic mental, or other psychotic disorder, with hospitalization history affecting priority status for housing eligibility. In addition, the difficulty in defining the mentally ill offender is compounded by the fact that frequently such individuals have multiple problems and can be diagnosed in multiple ways. For example, the mentally ill offender may also be mentally retarded or may have alcohol or drug addiction problems. This multiplicity of problems and possible diagnoses creates clear problems in accurately describing, understanding and responding to the population of mentally ill offenders. (p. 12)

DEVELOPING NEEDED MENTAL
HEALTH PROGRAMS FOR JAILS

DEVELOPING A COMPREHENSIVE MODEL

The initial step in establishing needed programming is the development of a comprehensive model. Figure 1 (p. 105) represents an overview of a comprehensive model, which will be described in detail in the sections that follow.

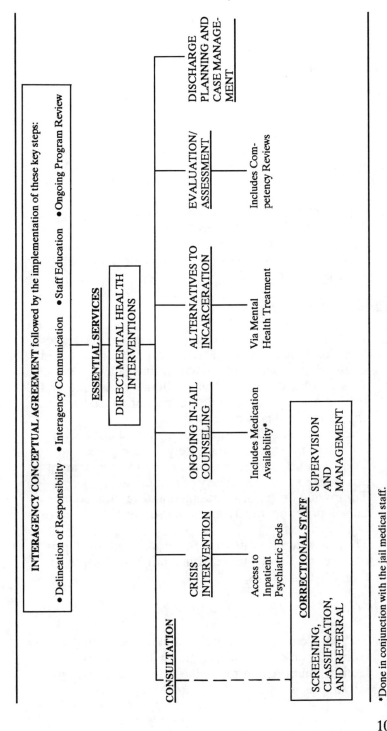

Figure 1. Comprehensive model of a mental health program for jails.

105

DEVELOPING A CONCEPTUAL AGREEMENT

Importance and Goals of the Conceptual Agreement. In light of the difficulties between the mental health and correctional systems, the establishment of a *joint conceptual agreement* is the foundation block of a collaborative jail mental health program. The chief administrators from the involved agencies need to reach agreement as to (a) *who will be served* by the program (target population), (b) the specific *goals* to be achieved by the program, and (c) the anticipated *consequences* for the target population, the staff, and the community for both achieving and not achieving the program goals.

An important initial step in the process of developing a conceptual agreement is defining goals. Based, partially, upon work done through the New York State Suicide Prevention Crisis Intervention Program, the following basic goals (Cox, Landsberg, & Paravati, 1989) are offered:

Client's Goals

1. To identify suicidal and seriously mentally ill inmates in a timely manner and provide for their care and safety within police lockups and county jails.
2. To significantly reduce the incidence of suicide and suicide attempts among persons incarcerated within county jails and police lockups.
3. To stabilize acutely mentally ill and/or suicidal prisoners and to provide for their safety.
4. To prevent decompensation among locally incarcerated prisoners with a history of mental illness.
5. To provide both non-sentenced and sentenced mentally ill prisoners timely access to appropriate levels of psychiatric care.
6. To provide continuity of care for all mentally ill prisoners upon their release from a jail or detention setting.

Staff Goals

1. To provide all jail and police lockup personnel with training and consultation that will enable them to identify, manage and refer suicidal and seriously mentally ill prisoners.

2. To provide all on-line mental health staff with an orientation to jail/lockup rules and regulations and to acquaint them with the unique challenges involved in dealing with the criminal justice system in general and with an incarcerated population in particular.

System Goals

1. To enhance coordination/communication between the criminal justice and mental health systems, thereby improving services and increasing both personal and agency accountability.
2. To provide local mental health authorities with practical operational guidelines that will enable them to implement or enhance crisis services for incarcerated persons.
3. To provide a realistic and cost effective model for the delivery of mental health care in jails and police lock-ups. (p. 104)

In addition to these specific goals, there is another key component of the conceptual agreement, namely: *Jails are community agencies and their clients (inmates) must be treated by community mental health providers.* Both the jail and the mental health system must acknowledge that the jails are a community resource and fall within the purview of a range of community agencies linked to the community mental health center.

To develop this conceptual agreement, high-level meetings of jail and community mental health agency representatives are essential. The mental health agency director, its high-level clinical staff, and the sheriff, warden, and key jail staff are essential participants.

DEFINING IMPLEMENTATION ISSUES

Delineation of Responsibilities. Based upon the conceptual agreement, it is essential to identify key areas of responsibility and then identify the type of personnel who will implement each responsibility. Table 1 (pp. 108-109) illustrates, in global terms, areas of activities and the type of personnel and agency with responsibility.

TABLE 1: SERVICE RESPONSIBILITIES

Service	Discipline	Program/Facility
Police Lockup		
Screening and Referral	Security	Police Lockup
Safety and Supervision	Security	Police Lockup
Emergency Outpatient Mental Health (MH) Services	Mental Health Medical	Local Hospital Emergency Room Clinic
Emergency Medical Services	Medical	Local Hospital Emergency Room
Psychiatric Inpatient Services	Mental Health	Local Hospital Psychiatric Inpatient Unit State Psychiatric Center
Consultation Services	Mental Health	Above Mental Health Programs
County Jail		
Screening and Referral	Security Medical	County Jail
Safety and Supervision	Security	County Jail
Emergency Outpatient Mental Health Services	Mental Health Medical	Local Hospital Emergency Room Clinic Other Emergency MH Service Program County Jail - Medical
Emergency Medical Services	Medical	County Jail - Medical General Hospital Emergency Room

Service	Discipline	Program/Facility
Psychiatric Inpatient Services	Mental Health	Local Hospital Psychiatric Inpatient Unit State Psychiatric Center
Consultation Services	Mental Health	Above Mental Health and Medical Programs

It is further recommended that, with regard to all areas of activity, jail/police and mental health agencies have detailed policies and procedures that will pinpoint responsibilities.

Interagency Communication. Regular ongoing interagency communication is a cornerstone for successful program implementation. This communication is necessary to insure:

- understanding of assigned roles and responsibilities;
- knowledge of each agency's capabilities and constraints;
- a continuing dialogue on programmatic implementation issues;
- needed care for specified clients; and
- appropriate response to crisis situations.

Staff Training for Mental Health and Correctional Staffs. Staff training for staffs of both mental health and correctional agencies is a critical component of the core model activities. Specifically, each training has different goals and objectives.

For correctional staff, the goals of training are as follows:

- to provide information on the roles and responsibilities with regard to the mentally ill inmate;
- to provide background information on mental health, mental retardation, and alcohol/substance abuse;
- to provide information to the officers to identify (a) the person who is undergoing a mental health crisis and may be at risk of suicide, and (b) the person who may be chronically mentally ill;

- to understand how, when, and where to access the mental care system; and
- to review the officer's role in managing and insuring the safety of the mentally ill inmate or the inmate at risk of suicide.

An effective correctional staff training program must be well organized and structured. The New York State Forensic Suicide Prevention/Crisis Intervention Model Training program, for instance, has an 8-hour didactic training program with defined educational modules, an interactive videotape, and accompanying educational materials (i.e., Officer's Handbook). The course is taught, jointly, by mental health professionals and correctional staff who have completed a "train the trainers" program.

For the mental health staff working in correctional settings, a similar structured training program is necessary. This training program provides:

- an overview of the Criminal Justice System with specific emphasis on the function of jails and police lockups;
- discussions on mental health interventions in jails and police lockups with emphasis on the scope and nature of the services to be provided, key environmental conditions (i.e., security scheduling) that affect service delivery, and the need for ongoing liaison with jail/lockup staff;
- a comprehensive overview of forensic laws within the state that affect key issues - psychiatric examinations, inpatient commitment, and possible options, including alternatives to incarceration; and
- the need for discharge planning for inmates to insure their linkage to mental health services upon their release from the correctional setting.

Ongoing Program Review. Ongoing program review consists of two types of activities: (a) scheduled (i.e., semiannual) formal meetings between mental health and jail lockup staffs, and (b) investigations and review meetings of untoward incidents, especially suicides. The scheduled meetings are essential to further formal communications and to examine program needs and directions. The investigations and review meetings of untoward incidents are also key and serve to (a) determine the contributing causes for the incident; (b) increase the accountability of jail and mental health staff for providing security and treatment, and (c) help address the emotional impact on staff of these incidents, especially suicide. Spellman and Heyne (1989), in discussing the "psychological autopsy for jail suicides," note that "the psychological autopsy should provide the opportunity for learning and emotional healing. . . . It assisted the staff in clarifying their feelings of loss and resulted in team building" (p. 174).

ESSENTIAL SERVICES OF CORRECTIONAL STAFF WITH MENTAL HEALTH STAFF CONSULTATION

Screening, Classification, and Referral. The task of screening, classification, and referral is the direct responsibility of the correctional staff. Yet, it is essential that there is continuing dialogue between the correctional and mental health staff on the design and implementation of the system in this area and ongoing consultation.

Screening for high-risk suicidal and seriously mentally ill inmates needs to be the fundamental component of the initial booking process at any correctional setting. The reason for the screening at intake is that *50% of suicides occur within the first 24 hours of admission to the jail*. Thus, immediate identification of the at-risk inmate is essential to a suicide prevention program. Intake is also the most appropriate and valued place to identify inmates who may be seriously mentally ill, but who are not suicidal. This identification "triggers" for the correctional system appropriate courses of action regarding housing, level of observation, and possible referral for specialized services.

Effective screening involves both face-to-face interviews and observational activities and should be initiated by a trained intake officer. To fulfill this task, numbers of municipalities and states have developed *Screening Guidelines*. An excellent example of such guidelines are those developed and utilized in the New York State Forensic Suicide Prevention Crisis Intervention Program. These Screening Guidelines, developed after an extensive review of the relevant literature and subject to intensive field testing, consist of data collected on high-risk factors (Morschauser & Sherman, 1989, pp. 116-120):

Identifying Data

- age
- sex

Emotional State

- Arresting/transporting officer believes detainee may be suicide risk.
- Detainee worried about nonlegal problems.
- Detainee is thinking about killing himself or herself.
- Detainee feels hopeless.
- Detainee shows signs of depression.
- Detainee appears overly anxious, afraid, or angry.
- Detainee feels unusually ashamed or embarrassed.
- Detainee acting and/or talking in a strange manner.
- Detainee has psychiatric history.

Alcohol and Substance Abuse

- Detainee has history of drug or alcohol abuse.
- Detainee is apparently under the influence of alcohol or drugs; if yes, is detainee showing signs of withdrawal or mental illness?

Suicide History

- Detainee has previous suicide attempt.
- Detainee's family or significant other has previous suicide attempt.

Local Support System

- Detainee lacks close family or friends.

Significant Loss

- Detainee has experienced significant loss within the last six months (job, death, divorce).
- Detainee holds position of respect in community and/or alleged crime is shocking in nature.

It has been demonstrated that the Screening Guidelines are easy to use (a trained officer can complete the form during the intake in approximately 8 minutes), and the instrument has proved quite valuable in identifying at-risk behaviors. Morschauser and Sherman (1989) comment on the value of the Screening Guidelines as follows:

> Repeated use of the screening form serves as an ongoing reminder of the need to be continuously cognizant of suicide risk. This daily use coupled with the increased knowledge of suicide resulting from training may have as significant an impact upon prevention as the formal results of screening. In addition, the effect of the Guidelines is to focus the staff's attention to suicide risk. (p. 132)

Screening needs to be followed up by *classification*, which leads to determinations of housing and the level of supervision required. Suicidal or seriously mentally ill inmates may be assigned to special holding/observation cells or even in medical tiers, depending on the availability or lack of it within a given jail setting. Classification will also determine the required level of supervision of the inmate, which is discussed below. The screening can and may lead to referral to the mental health staff either for crisis intervention or for further evaluation and ongoing treatment.

Supervision and Management. The supervision of inmates is a responsibility of the correctional agency. Based upon the initial screening described earlier and the mental health-jail/lockup staff communication, key levels of supervision will include *constant observation*, observed continuously; *close observation*, observed every 15 minutes; or *regular supervision*, observed every 30 minutes. Management decisions (e.g., removal of potentially dangerous objects) are also part of this ongoing dialogue.

Liability Issues. In developing jail suicide prevention/crisis intervention programs, both for the jail and for the mental health agency, there exists the potential issue of liability. Actually, for the jail, the potential of liability suits exists whether it has a suicide prevention program or not. Yet, in fact, the jail, in having a suicide prevention program with appropriate screening, classification, and management procedures administered by a trained jail staff and with linkages to mental health agencies, significantly reduces its potential liability. The mental health agency, in offering services to the jails for screening and treating "at-risk inmates," increases its potential liability. Lawsuits in the case of successful suicides may not be directed only at the jail and its staff, but may also be directed at the mental health agency and its staff. However, realistically, this should not be of substantial concern to the mental health agency. Courts have generally recognized that it is not possible to identify and prevent all jail suicides. Rather, courts have focused on cases where there are overt and obvious signs of suicidal behavior in the inmate and where the institution generally neglected to take any, even minimal, actions to protect the safety of that inmate.

DIRECT MENTAL HEALTH
SERVICES PROVIDED TO JAILS

Crisis Intervention. Crisis intervention is the key essential service provided by mental health agencies to jails/lockups. This crisis intervention service should be available 24 hours a day and 7 days a week.

It should ideally include the availability for mental health professional staff to go to the jail/police lockup to examine the inmate and, in consultation with correctional staff, decide on appropriate actions. The possible actions include:

1. Stabilization within the jail/lockup setting. (This may require use of psychotropic medication; the availability of physicians/psychiatrists to assist in this process is essential. The responsibility of prescribing and the administering of psychotropic medications may vary depending upon the agreement between the mental health team and the jail health service, that is, it can be done by the physician/nurse in the jail medical service or by the psychiatrist/clinician on the mental health team.
2. Removal to an emergency room or psychiatric emergency room for further evaluation, medical treatment, or alternate disposition.
3. Transfer to a psychiatric inpatient service.

For a crisis intervention service to be effective, it must have access to inpatient psychiatric beds. This may require multiple agency agreements or networks and may not be easily achieved in light of the reluctance of some psychiatric inpatient services to treat inmates. Yet, this is essential. In rural counties, without local community-based inpatient psychiatric beds or psychiatric emergency services, alternative arrangements, through agreements with state psychiatric centers, will be needed.

Also of fundamental importance to a crisis intervention service is the ability to work actively with the inmate if he or she is stabilized in the correctional facility. This may necessitate numerous visits over short periods of time to work with the specific inmate. Finally, a key component of a crisis intervention service is continuing communication and consultation with the correctional staff.

Evaluation and Assessment. Evaluation and assessment are important services of a mental health agency to a jail/lockup. The type of services provided can and should include:

1. Competency evaluations (formal evaluations for the court to determine the individual's competency to stand trial).
2. Assessment of an individual's functional disorder to assist the court/criminal justice system in determination of actions.
3. Ability to evaluate developmental disability issues. (Increasing numbers of the mentally retarded/developmentally disabled are becoming involved in the criminal justice system.)

It is important to note these evaluations to the court only as "recommendations" by an outside consultant. In the court system, the judge, district attorney, or the defendant's attorney can seek additional "expert psychiatric opinions." Further, it is up to the judge to formally decide how to utilize the assessment of the mental health staff in his or her ultimate decision making.

Ongoing In-Jail Counseling. Ideally, the mental health agency should be able to provide ongoing in-jail mental health counseling programs. This can involve several different approaches:

1. Individual counseling.
2. Group therapy (it has been indicated that target group therapy activities - e.g., for groups of alcoholics; for drug abusers; for child abusers - can be an important vehicle for initiating treatment).
3. Family support interventions (work with families, while the inmate is detained, is frequently helpful to improve

the inmate's interest in pursuing further treatment after discharge and maintaining a stable family environment).

Ongoing counseling in the jail can be provided to inmates at any stage of their incarceration (pretrial or posttrial). They should only be provided based upon a joint assessment of needs by jail and mental health personnel.

Discharge Planning and Case Management. Planning for the release of the mentally ill inmate is essential, if he or she is to be maintained and stabilized in the community. The postrelease planning should begin as early as possible in the inmate's detention period to provide continuity to complete necessary arrangements for ongoing treatment and support services. The need for linkage of the inmate to the mental health agency is *essential.* The mental health staff, working in the jail, need to arrange for a specific appointment within several days after release. It may be necessary to have mental health staff accompany the former inmate to his or her first appointment or appointments. Involvement of the family is also useful to reinforce the need and importance of ongoing treatment.

As important as treatment is, the need for case management is also critical. Case management to find the dischargee needed residential, financial, medical, training, and other services has been demonstrated to be an extremely effective tool (Borgman, 1975). Case management may also be significant in assisting the former inmate to establish and maintain his or her relationship with parole/probation authorities, if they are involved. Finally, it needs to be understood that to achieve the maximum potential of keeping the mentally ill client out of continuing involvement with the criminal justice system, intensive and ongoing clinical intervention and case management may be required.

Mental Health Treatment as an Alternative to Incarceration. For the mentally ill offender, mental health treatment and support can be an alternative to incarceration. Interest in this approach has increased over the past several years. Based upon review and observation, there appear to be two approaches to the use of mental health treatment as an alternative to incarceration. The first, and more common, approach is an informal strategy in which mental health intervention teams in jails/lockups will, on a case-by-case basis, arrange for treatment alternatives to jail. The second approach is a more formal systematic strategy of developing specific diversion programs.

With respect to the first, more widespread approach, the example of experiences at Ulster County Mental Health Services in Kingston, New York, is illustrative. Ulster County Mental Health Services, serving a small (160,000 population) rural county midway between New York City and Albany, provides extensive services to a 120-bed county jail. The mental health treatment team identified inmates who, in terms of the pending charge and presenting problems, would be more appropriately served by a mental health inpatient, residential, or outpatient treatment rather than by incarceration. Team members worked with the defense lawyers, the district attorney's office staff, and judges and arranged for disposition to other facilities. Frequently, the dispositions were to state psychiatric facilities, facilities for the developmentally disabled, acute inpatient units, and, occasionally, outpatient services. In all cases, the mental health team members followed the cases to insure that, upon return to the community, needed treatment and residential care services were available. In a 15-month period between April, 1986, and July, 1987, the team treated 164 clients and was able to assist 45 to be transferred to treatment services (Landsberg, 1987).

A more formal and systematic approach is described by Sagner (1985) in a paper entitled "Keeping the Mentally Ill Out of Jail: The Milwaukee Approach." This approach serves as a diversion for chronically mentally ill:

> The program employs methods which are effective in dealing with unmotivated and resistive, sometimes openly hostile and excessively acting out chronic mentally ill [CMI] clients. It is designed to work with the "hard core" CMI who have extensive treatment histories and who do poorly in treatment because they fail to stay in treatment or follow treatment directions. The program utilizes the usual medical, psychiatric and intensive case approach. It also makes extensive use of incentives and rewards as well as the more authoritarian use of leverage available through the criminal justice system. It uses methods which are clearly designed to keep the client in treatment and induce changes of behavior and lifestyle along more constructive lines. (p. 4)

The key elements of the program are:

(1) Provision of basic needs for the client - food, shelter, clothing, medical care - which are provided on the first day of the client's involvement with the program.
(2) Provision of intensive treatment, including medication, of up to 5 days a week.
(3) Use of financial incentives. The program serves as the payor of the client's income/benefits. Money is budgeted and distributed regularly to clients. (Sagner, 1985, p. 2)

A detailed research report on the effectiveness of mental health treatment as an alternative to incarceration based upon a North Carolina program indicated the following:

*Nearly 1/2 (19 of 39 clients) "appear to have ceased law violating behaviors"
*The most effective interventions appear to be:
    -community mental health agency treatment alone
    -state psychiatric hospitalizations followed by community treatment
*The least effective treatment was state hospitalizations alone
*Successful intervention requires:
    -mutual agreement between the treatment agency and the client as to the problem that needs to be addressed
    -acknowledging that these clients may be psychologically immature
    -the provision of case management services (Borgman, 1975, p. 425)

CAUTIONARY NOTES

In the materials just presented, an extensive program of mental health services was described. Implementation of the full program may be beyond the scope of any agency or network of agencies or a locality. The specific programs developed within localities must be targeted toward that community. To this end, collaboration between the jail and mental health agencies is essential in developing the specific plan for that community. Additionally, it should be recognized that the specific programs developed for rural counties may be significantly different than those in more populated areas. Within rural areas, different types of options (e.g., three-way agreements between the jail, the community mental health agency, and the state psychiatric centers) may be required. Agencies/communities should *not* feel constrained to implement the model as described.

STRATEGIES FOR RESOURCE DEVELOPMENT

Developing needed mental health services in jails requires appropriate resources available for the mental health agency. The agency administrator and clinical staff must initially assess whether the agency within its existing manpower can reassign needed staff to a jail mental health program or can expand the scope of an existing service (e.g., the crisis intervention program) to adequately serve the jail. To the extent that existing resources/programs can be refocused to serve the jail, the less need for the agency to seek additional financial resources.

It does seem likely that numerous mental health agencies will need additional financial resources to develop jail services. If these resources are needed, it is essential that the mental health agency work collaboratively with the jail so that the institution becomes its ally in the quest for funds. The search for funds should encompass several strategies and directions:

1. Seeking traditional mental health funding

    a. through the state - by identifying the possible number of the chronically mentally ill that can be served;
    b. through the locality - by emphasizing the importance of mental health treatment in suicide prevention programs and alternatives to incarceration efforts and pinpointing potential financial benefits that can result; and
    c. through grants for pilot programs and activities.

2. Seeking criminal justice services funding

    a. by having the jail, through funds they may have, be able to purchase services from the mental health agency; and
    b. via funding sources for alternative incarceration programs.

119

The availability of funding may vary significantly by state and locality and will have a significant impact on the scope of the program developed.

CONCLUSIONS

The future holds dramatically little hope other than that the jails will continue to be the institution of last resort for the mentally ill and "will continue to incarcerate individuals needing mental health services" (McCarty, Steadman, & Morrissey, 1982, p. 56). The reasons for this continued trend are (Craig & Kissel, 1988):

- an unlikelihood that policies or procedures for state mental hospitalizations will drastically change; and
- society's continued intolerance of mentally disordered behavior and the use of the criminal justice system to resolve or remove the problem.

Thus, it is imperative that, for effective planning and service delivery to occur, jails and local community mental health agencies must establish cordial and extensive relationships.

As previously noted, the key element in developing needed programming is the establishment of an interagency conceptual agreement. This agreement should provide a clear direction for the program and should identify client, staff, and system goals. Accompanying this agreement should be a delineation of responsibilities, interagency communication, staff training, and program review activities. Program development should then focus on consultation to correctional staff to assist them with their fundamental tasks of screening, classification, and referral and for supervision and management. The actual mental health programming, if possible, should include crisis intervention (including access to inpatient psychiatric care), evaluation/assessment services, ongoing in-jail counseling, postjail discharge planning (including case management), and alternatives to incarceration. If comprehensive programming is not possible due to funding difficulties, then the focus should be on crisis intervention and ongoing consultation.

Jails and community mental health agencies share common ground - the mentally ill incarcerated client. Thus, it is essential that we work together to address their needs.

Gerald Landsberg, DSW, MPA, is currently Chairman of the Social Welfare Programs and Policies at the New York University Graduate School of Social Work, New York. He formerly served as Assistant Commissioner for Strategic Planning in the New York City Department of Mental Health, Mental Retardation, and Alcoholism Services and was co-chair of the New York State Office of Mental Health Forensic Task Force. He co-edited two editions of the *Psychiatric Quarterly* devoted to jail suicides, and has authored or co-authored several articles and chapters on forensic issues. Dr. Landsberg may be contacted at New York University School of Social Work, 3 Washington Square North, New York, NY 10003.

REFERENCES

Atlas, R. (1989, Summer). Reducing the opportunity for inmate suicide: A design guide. *Psychiatric Quarterly, 60,* 161-172.

Bogira, S. (1981, April 10). Psych team. *Chicago Reader,* pp. 1-52.

Bolton, A. (1976). *A Study of the Need for an Availability of Mental Health Services for Mentally Disordered Jail Inmates and Juveniles in Detention Facilities.* Sacramento, CA: California Department of Health.

Borgman, R. (1975, July). Diversion of law violators to mental health facilities. *Social Casework,* pp. 418-426.

Brodsky, S. (1987, September 27-29). *Intervention Models for Mental Health Services in Jails.* National Workshop on Mental Health Services in Jails, Baltimore, MD.

Burtch, B. E., & Ericson, R. V. (1979). *The Silent System: An Inquiry into Prisoners Who Suicide and Annotated Bibliography.* Toronto: University of Toronto, Center of Criminology.

Callahan, L. A., & Diamond, R. J. (1985). *Mad, Bad or Both? A Survey of the Mentally Ill in Jail.* Madison, WI: University of Wisconsin.

Chaiklin, H. (1986, March 19). *Current and Prior Mental Health Treatment of Jail Inmates - The Jail as an Alternative Shelter.* Annual Meeting of the Academy of Criminal Justice, Orlando, FL.

Charle, S. (1981, August). Suicide in the cellblocks: New programs attack the No. 1 killer of jail inmates. *Correction Magazine,* pp. 6-16.

Cox, J., Landsberg, G., & Paravati, P. (1989, Summer). Essential components of a forensic suicide crisis intervention program. *Psychiatric Quarterly, 60,* 103-118.

Cox, J., McCarty, D., Landsberg, G., & Paravati, P. (1989, Winter). A model for crisis intervention services in the jails. *International Journal of Law and Psychiatry, 11,* 391-407.

Craig, R., & Kissel, M. (1988, August). The mentally ill offender: Punishment or treatment. *State Legislative Report, 11*(13).

Danto, B. (Ed.). (1973). *Jail House Blues: A Study of Suicidal Behavior in Jails and Prisons.* Orchard Lake, MI: Epic Publications.

Detention Reporter. (1986, April).

Hayes, L. M. (1989, Spring). National study of jail suicides . . . Seven years later. *Psychiatric Quarterly, 160,* 7-30.

Landsberg, G. (1987, August). *Mental Health Services in the Ulster County Jail.* Unpublished paper.

Massachusetts Department of Mental Health. (1980). Unpublished report.

Massachusetts Special Commission to Investigate Suicides in Municipal Detention Centers. (1984). *Suicides in Massachusetts Lockup 1973-1984.* Boston, MA: Author.

McCarty, D., Steadman, H. J., & Morrissey, J. (1982). Issues in planning jail mental health services. *Federal Probation, 46,* 56-63.

Morrissey, J., Steadman, H. J., Kilburn, H., & Lindsay, M. (1984, June). The effectiveness of jail mental health programs: An interorganizational assessment. *Criminal Justice & Behavior, 11,* 235-256.

Morschauser, P., & Sherman, L. (1989, Summer). The New York State Suicide Survey Guidelines. *Psychiatric Quarterly, 60,* 115-134.

National Center on Institutions and Alternatives. (1981). *And Darkness Closes in . . . National Study of Jail Suicides.* Alexandria, VA: Author.

National Coalition for Jail Reform. (1984). *Removing the Chronically Mentally Ill from Jail.* Washington, DC: Author.

National Institute of Corrections. (1983). *Suicide in Jails.* Boulder, CO: Correction Information Center.

New York State Office of Mental Health. (1986a). *Local Forensic Suicide Prevention Crisis Intervention Program.* Albany, NY: Author.

New York State Office of Mental Health. (1986b). *Mental Health Information Handbook.* Albany, NY: Author.

New York State Office of Mental Health. *Forensic Task Force Report.* (1991). Albany, NY: Author.

New York State Office of Mental Health and the New York State Commission on Corrections. (1986). *Policy and Procedural Guidelines Manual for County Correctional Facilities.* Albany, NY: NYSOMH.

Sagner, B. (1985, November 14). *The Milwaukee Approach.* Presentation at the American Correctional Health Care Association Annual Meeting, Chicago, IL.

Shinn, E. (1987). *Analysis of the New York State Suicide Prevention Screening Guidelines.* Unpublished report.

Spellman, A., & Heyne, B. (1989, Summer). Psychological autopsy. *Psychiatric Quarterly, 60,* 173-184.

Steadman, H. J., & Morrissey, J. (1978). The arrest rates of mental patients and criminal offenders. *American Journal of Psychiatry, 138.*

Steadman, H. J., & Ribner, S. A. (1980). Changing perceptions of the mental health needs of inmates in local jails. *American Journal of Psychiatry, 137,* 1115-1116.

Teplin, L. (1984, July). Criminalizing mental disorders: The comparative arrest rate of the mentally ill. *American Psychologist, 39,* 794-803.

Teplin, L., Filstead, W., Hefter, G., & Sheridan, E. (1980, May). Police involvement with the psychiatric emergency patient. *Psychiatric Annals, 10,* 203-207.

Valdiserri, E., Carroll, K., & Hartl, A. (1986, February). A study of offenses committed by psychotic inmates in a county jail. *Hospital and Community Psychiatry, 37,* 163-166.

6

Changing Roles: Psychiatry in Community Mental Health Centers

David A. Pollack and David L. Cutler

The goal of this chapter is to describe the role of the psychiatrist in community mental health programs, emphasizing the historical trends leading to the current state of psychiatric practice in community mental health centers (CMHCs). The chapter contains an analysis of psychiatry in community mental health programs with descriptions of the types of roles psychiatrists play and their feelings about those roles. The following sections focus on the ways psychiatrists can be trained and utilized in community mental health programs so that both the psychiatrist and the agency benefit and are satisfied. Recommendations for ways psychiatrists can succeed in community mental health practice and for methods that mental health administrators can successfully use to recruit and retain psychiatrists conclude the chapter.

HISTORY OF PSYCHIATRISTS'
ROLES IN COMMUNITY MENTAL HEALTH

The theoretical basis for community mental health practice began with the seminal work of several psychiatrists. Eric Lindemann (1944) defined the stages of grief and a method for intervening in the grief process to prevent depression. Gerald Caplan, however, was the most important early theoretician in community psychiatry. His book, *Principles of Preventive Psychiatry* (1963), formed the basis for community mental health concepts of the 1960s and 1970s and is still in use today. George Engel (1982) formulated the "biopsychosocial model," to which most community psychiatrists now adhere. In addition, countless psychiatrists have provided major leadership in program development and clinical practice since the early days of the community mental health movement. It would be hard to imagine community mental health without direct service and advocacy from psychiatrists. This, of course, was also true in the 19th century during the state hospital movement and in the early 20th century with the mental hygiene movement.

Beginning with the 1963 Community Mental Health Center Act (Public Law 88-164) and staffing amendments of 1965, over 700 mental health centers were eventually financed and built. This was accomplished by using federal mental health center grants that provided seed money matched with local funds, with the federal funds phased out over a 5- to 8-year period. In the 1960s and 1970s many of these centers were established and administered by psychiatrists. However, during the decade of the 1970s the relative presence of full-time equivalent (FTE) psychiatrists in community mental health centers decreased dramatically. For example, between 1970 and 1973 the number of FTEs in CMHCs decreased from 6.8 to 4.5 (Bass, 1978). Since then, that number has dropped to less than four FTEs per mental health center (Dewey & Astrachan, 1985).

Although the absolute numbers of psychiatrists increased over the years, they were spread over a decreasing number of FTEs. Psychiatrists more frequently were asked to provide direct care, but not training, supervision, consultation, and administrative work. At the same time, caseloads were changing. The numbers of patients served per full-time equivalent psychiatrist per center more than doubled (from 347 to 731 patients per FTE) between 1974 and 1979. Unfortunately, the degree of disability and complexity of the clinical disorders of these patients increased steadily during the same period of time (Pardes, Pincus, & Pomeranz, 1985).

As community mental health programs became financially more complex, psychiatrists became disenchanted with, and lost interest in, administrative work. They appeared increasingly ill equipped to be administrators, and their training provided minimal support to develop such skills. Other clinicians and administrators experienced frustration and disappointment about psychiatrists' difficulties or failures as administrators. Often nonmedical staff expressed resentment and jealousy toward psychiatrist-administrators, who received disproportionately higher salaries than nonmedical administrators. When psychiatrists were placed in supervisory roles, they often were perceived as intruders whose medical perspective was felt to be unnecessary and even alien instead of supportive to the psychotherapy and social service mission of the clinic staff (Peterson, 1981).

In 1971 more than half of the community mental health centers were headed by psychiatrist-administrators. By 1980 the number of psychiatrist-administrators declined to less than 20%, and by 1985 still fewer (8%) administrators were psychiatrists (Knox, 1985). Replacing them were mostly social workers and psychologist executive directors. However, in some instances they were replaced by executives who had no significant clinical training or background. Among these nonclinician administrators have been lawyers, public administrators, members of the clergy, or budget analysts, whose main focus often was fiscal management instead of clinical leadership and support (Talbott, 1979).

CURRENT STATUS OF PSYCHIATRISTS
IN COMMUNITY MENTAL HEALTH

What is the current state of psychiatry in CMHC settings? How are psychiatrists spending their time? How do they feel about their roles?

Very few psychiatrists are involved in administration, supervision, consultation, or training in community mental health centers. There is a small pool of psychiatrists who are adequately trained to function as administrators. Diamond et al. (1985) have identified a number of issues related to training that may have reduced the number of psychiatrists available and adequately trained for this type of practice. These include the following:

1. Psychiatry is often less valued as a medical discipline by medical students.
2. Public psychiatric work is often less valued by psychiatric residents.
3. There are few psychiatric residency training programs in public facilities.
4. Social and community psychiatry training programs are few in number and sometimes not very well organized. They often must compete with other aspects of psychiatric training programs.
5. There are too few academic psychiatrists who are capable of adequately teaching community mental health princi-

ples and practice. Those psychiatrists who are capable are
often not found in academic settings, but instead are
working in community mental health programs.

6. There are numerous systems issues, such as conflicting
   missions within the training facility, bureaucratic red tape,
   geographic barriers to getting trainees to public training
   sites, and weak links between psychiatric training programs and public sector mental health programs.
7. Finally, there are other issues relating to values conflicts,
   socio-political factors, and economic conditions.

With fewer dollars available, especially during the Reagan era
when social services suffered cutbacks, mental health administra
tors have narrowed the role of psychiatrists. The emphasis has
shifted to increased direct service. The psychiatrist's time is clearly the most expensive, and there is an incentive to keep it to a
minimum. The result is that psychiatrists are frequently limited
to performing the tasks that are unquestionably and unambigu-
ously those which only a physician can do. The emphasis here is
on *physician* more than on psychiatrist, because those tasks are
primarily ones of prescribing medications, ordering lab tests,
evaluating for side effects, medical screening, and signing documents, such as insurance forms or treatment plans, that only a
physician can sign.

The growth of other mental health disciplines, such as social
work, psychology, and psychiatric nursing has increased the pool
of less expensive personnel. Mental health administrators perceive these professionals as able to perform tasks that previously
only psychiatrists could perform. Thus, nonpsychiatrist mental
health professionals have increasingly assumed supervisory, consultative, and training positions in CMHCs.

The shortage of social service dollars has pushed some administrators to eliminate many nonreimbursable activities. Since the
early 1980s, mental health centers have begun to shift from a
general comprehensive approach to one more focused on specific
target populations. States have developed community support
programs emphasizing the treatment of severe and chronically
mentally ill (CMI) persons. Performance contracts have become
the preferred mode of funding services in many states. The need
to meet contract goals based on units of direct services to clients
has blurred the value of nonbillable activities, especially in the
eyes of administrators, who are pressured to focus on costs and
revenues. Thus, consultation, supervision, and training have

come to be seen as luxuries, as nonessential activities, or as potentially supportive activities that programs regretfully have to cut or cannot reinstate because of their expense and lack of visible (i.e., fiscal) value.

In recent years, as case management has become the basic activity that mental health centers provide, many bachelor's level persons have begun to occupy positions that previously were taken up by social workers with higher levels of training. The result of this trend is a partial deprofessionalization process. Unfortunately, the further this process progresses, the less likely psychiatrists are to be as heavily involved. This occurs at a time when more patients have little access to state hospitals but require more intensive treatment because they (a) take medications that cause significant side effects, (b) have numerous complicating medical problems, or (c) are using addictive substances to escape their misery.

Many mental health centers are poorly equipped to deal with these problems. Frequently, health clinics and private physicians are not willing to take patients who are covered by welfare or social security disability. State governments try to get increasingly more work with fewer and decreasing resources. Staff have very little time to do anything but track their patients and keep up with paper work, and they are often unwilling or unable to use psychiatrists as consultants or supervisors. For whatever reason, a major effect of these changes has been to de-emphasize the role of psychiatrists in mental health centers. This is a major loss of grace for a profession that was largely responsible for spawning the movement in the first place. The situation then becomes very frustrating and, for many good psychiatrists, simply not acceptable. As a result they escape to the private sector, often regretting that bureaucratic or other factors prevented them from serving the community.

For those who remain in community mental health programs, many are faced with the prototypical worst-case scenario of the psychiatrist's role, which some people have dubbed the "giant in the closet" syndrome. This "giant" is the part-time contract psychiatrist who is restricted to seeing patients for diagnostic evaluations, prescribing medications, and signing necessary insurance and treatment documents. It is not uncommon for a psychiatrist to be asked to sign such forms for patients seen only once or not at all by the psychiatrist - in effect to "rubber stamp" approval of the primary clinician's work without significant psychiatric involvement. The psychiatrist who is compliant and provides medicine and signatures whenever someone asks is seen as a "good doctor." The psychiatrist who asks questions may be seen as a "troublemaker." Such a psychiatrist is not integrated into the center, is not respected with regard to the management of cases, and is seen as a "necessary evil" whose presence, although unwanted, is required for reimbursement and accountability purposes (Peterson, 1981).

Somewhere lost in these unfortunate dynamics is the idea that the psychiatrist is a very broadly trained generalist who can provide support and supervision to a wide range of clinicians working in community mental health programs. In its place is the attitude that there are many prescriptions to be written and the only one who can perform this function is the doctor, while the remaining mental health treatment functions can be provided by less expensive nonpsychiatrist clinicians. The biopsychosocial model has been either abandoned or substantially discounted.

Vaccaro and Clark (1987), through a survey of psychiatrists in public practice, assessed the level of psychiatrists' satisfaction with their roles in community mental health programs (Clark & Vaccaro, 1987; Vaccaro & Clark, 1987). Among the areas of dissatisfaction reported by many psychiatrists are (a) lack of support from administrators; (b) lack of validation from and value to other staff; (c) low pay; (d) responsibility without authority; (e) pressure to sign documents on patients who are unknown to the psychiatrist; (f) decreased variety of tasks, and lack of stimulation; (g) professional isolation; (h) work overload; (i) unpleasant working conditions; and (j) internal politics and staff conflict.

The growing concern among community psychiatrists regarding their role conflicts, dissatisfactions, and lack of professional identity led to the formation of The American Association of Community Psychiatrists and to attempts to develop minimum standards or guidelines for psychiatric practice within community mental health programs. These standards (Clark, 1988) describe the specific roles that may be appropriate for such positions as medical director and staff psychiatrist in a CMHC. They also clarify the psychiatrist's level of authority, the meaning of the psychiatrist's signature, and the nature of the psychiatrist's supervisory relationship with other clinicians in the center.

SUCCESSFUL ROLE MODELS

In spite of the extensive number of problems cited in the Vaccaro and Clark (1987) study, many of which are serious role conflicts, most of the psychiatrists report significant overall satisfaction with their community mental health jobs - sufficient satisfaction that the vast majority of respondents had spent more than 4 years in their CMHCs. This seems to indicate that, for many community psychiatrists, positive factors such as (a) doing meaningful community service for disadvantaged patients, (b) variety of work, (c) collegiality and teamwork, and (d) financial and work schedule security often outweigh the negatives.

What may be more meaningful about this survey is the notion that some hard-working psychiatrists (who may hardly be known outside their own communities) have succeeded in creating roles for themselves that are satisfying and mutually beneficial to them, their patients, their colleagues and supervisees, and the agency as a whole.

Diamond et al. (1985) identified three categories of psychiatrists who work in community mental health centers: recent graduates or relocating physicians who take part-time work while establishing a private practice; private practice psychiatrists who provide part-time service to community mental health centers out of a commitment to public psychiatry; and those who "out of enthusiasm, special training, or plain stubbornness, pursue a long-term career in community mental health" (p. 34).

Although the potential for satisfaction and success in public practice may be correlated with the types of practice categorized previously, it may more likely be linked to factors specific to the psychiatrist, the training the psychiatrist receives, and the organization for which the psychiatrist works (Faulkner et al., 1982). We will describe one training program that has tried to address these issues.

PUBLIC PSYCHIATRY TRAINING IN OREGON

Community psychiatry training in Oregon has evolved since 1973 and is now called the "Public Psychiatry Training Program." It is integrated into the general psychiatric residency and involves three major blocks of time: in the second year for state hospital, the third year community, and the fourth year administrative training. The program is administered by a board made up of representatives of the state mental health division, the state hospitals, the community mental health centers directors organization, the dean of the medical school, and the chairman of the department of psychiatry (Cutler, Bloom, & Shore, 1981; Shore, Kinzie, & Bloom, 1979). These individuals oversee the program to assure that psychiatrists are trained to meet the needs for public psychiatrists in Oregon. This includes both state hospitals and mental health centers.

In the third year of training all residents are asked to select a rotation at a community mental health center anywhere in the state of Oregon. Residents browse through an agency profile notebook that contains information on all of the mental health agencies in the state and then discuss their observations with the director or associate director of the Public Psychiatry Training Program. They are asked to visit two or three of these programs prior to beginning their rotation. They then select which program they wish to be placed in and begin a 6-month, half-time rotation in community psychiatry.

During the first 6 weeks the residents are encouraged to survey the program by visiting all the service elements and subcontract agencies. They then negotiate a work contract. This rotation is accompanied by the Public Psychiatry seminar. This interdisciplinary seminar includes master's degree nursing students who also have community placements, and focuses to a large extent on the care of the chronically mentally ill and other special populations as well as on mental health consultation skills. Residents receive supervision by staff of the Public Psychiatry Training Program and on-site supervision at the mental health center. Residents are encouraged to work collaboratively with agency staff. They are never allowed to spend more than 50% of their time seeing patients, so that they have adequate time to get involved in other kinds of activities that go on in the mental health center, such as administration, quality assurance, supervision and training, and mental health consultation outside the agency. By the end of this rotation residents are expected to have the following skills and attitudes:

A. Skills - The ability to:

1. Enter a community mental health delivery system with a clear understanding of the psychiatrist's role;
2. Distinguish between levels of intervention and prevention;
3. Perform case management (assessment, planning, linking, monitoring, and advocacy);
4. Plan, work, and relate on an interdisciplinary team for the provision of direct or indirect services for long-term mentally disabled persons;

    5. Negotiate a consultation contract;
    6. Conduct a mental health consultation with a community agency;
    7. Initiate basic mental health program planning strategies;
    8. Work through a process of consultation termination;
    9. Conduct precommitment evaluation and court examinations under the state's commitment statute; and
  10. Demonstrate a thorough understanding of the use of medications in collaboration with nonmedical staff with special regard to compliance and informed consent.

B. Attitudes:

    1. Appropriate respect and sensitivity to racial, cultural, and ethnic values of patients, families, and interdisciplinary mental health team members;
    2. Responsibility to patients, their families, and significant others, including agency people, and appropriate respect for their opinions and welfare;
    3. Willingness to consider and evaluate criticism and peer review of one's professional work;
    4. Commitment to evaluation of treatment results as based on established methods;
    5. Comfort in dealing with highly personal and emotionally charged situations; and
    6. Sensitivity to and willingness to explore a variety of opinions and attitudes and ideas set forth by patients, patient advocates, and community people at large.

In the fourth year residents have an opportunity to spend a full year working in an intensive specialty clinic with long-term mentally ill patients or to take an elective within the mental health division that focuses on long-term patients. This could include an elective in administrative psychiatry focusing on the chronically mentally ill, an elective in forensic psychiatry, or an elective in state hospital specialty units. Clinical electives in psychiatric rehabilitation are available and are based at rehabilitation-oriented day treatment programs. The University Hospital Outpatient Clinic includes two specialty clinics that focus on CMI. For the fourth year administrative elective, residents are supervised by the director of the Public Psychiatry Training

Program and either the director of programs for the mentally and emotionally disturbed for the state or by the administrator of the state mental health division. This intensive supervision in the fourth year allows residents to be in contact with psychiatrists who play major administrative and program planning roles. They receive first-hand experience in public mental health planning and administrative activities. The state mental health division, by law, must focus most of its energy on the chronically mentally ill. Residents have the opportunity to see how the planning process works within a value system that is dedicated to the public patient. They work side by side with staff of the Division and consultants from the Public Psychiatry Training Program doing research, planning, and site visits for the Division throughout the state.

EXAMPLES OF SUCCESSFUL COMMUNITY PSYCHIATRISTS

To demonstrate some psychiatrist-linked qualities it may be useful to describe actual examples of community psychiatrists who have developed successful roles for themselves.

Example 1. For the past 6 years, since he completed his residency training, Dr. A has been working as a team psychiatrist on a multidisciplinary case management (community support) team in a large urban CMHC. His half-time position includes direct care responsibility for approximately 130 chronically mentally ill patients. He does initial psychiatric diagnostic evaluations on all patients, prescribes medications, and reviews and supervises treatment planning, all as an integrated member of the team. He participates in administrative activities, including regular medical staff meetings and a committee to develop policies, programmatic services, and training for staff and clients on AIDS-related issues. He has teaching opportunities and chairs a weekly clinical case conference. In addition to this job he works at another CMHC for less time and has a small private practice.

Example 2. Dr. B, who has a thriving private practice in a rural community, has been working for approximately 1 day per week at the area community mental health program for the past 15 years. Her long-term training and consulting relationship with the agency has led to a very high level of staff expertise regarding psychiatric diagnosis, the use of medications, and strategies for

134

effectively working with relatively noncompliant chronic mental patients. Her emphasis on training and collaborative approaches to patients has helped to prevent splitting by patients and has fostered the mutual development of staff self-confidence and trust between staff and the psychiatrist.

Example 3. Dr. C works four-fifths time in a rural county mental health program. He provides training and supervision to what is largely a paraprofessional staff. He has responsibility for programs for the severe and chronically mentally ill. The director and staff of the program have known him since his placement there as a resident in the community psychiatry training program. They have indicated that his work has been excellent and that they could not get along without him. He is a dedicated public psychiatrist, but the program has had great difficulty in finding adequate funds to pay him. As a result, his morale had been low. He considered leaving, but changed his mind when a more suitable agreement was reached to compensate him at a more reasonable level.

Example 4. Dr. D works four-fifths time in a blended position as medical director of a large downtown urban community mental health center and as a public psychiatry training program faculty member at a university medical center. Her CMHC roles are varied, including hiring and administrative supervision of medical staff, clinical consultation to a shelter for homeless mentally ill, ad hoc consultation (clinical troubleshooting) to all agency programs as backup to the various staff psychiatrists, training for clinic staff, psychiatric consultation to primary care providers in nearby community health clinics, policy and procedure development and oversight for a wide range of quality assurance activities, and participation in various levels of overall management at the agency. She is active in state mental health division activities, such as a mental health advisory board and a task force to develop rules regarding minimum standards for community mental health program clinical records.

CONCLUSIONS AND
RECOMMENDATIONS

Why are the preceding psychiatrists successful and relatively satisfied with their public activities? It would seem that certain factors that are essential to one's survival as a community psychiatrist are present in all of these examples. Of course, it helps to be able to work with enlightened, sensitive, and gifted administrators and with talented and committed staff, both of which are found in many centers across the country. But there are psychiatrist-linked factors that could be summarized as follows:

1. There should be a commitment to serving the community with secondary regard to personal monetary gain, although remuneration should be sufficient to make community work attractive.
2. It is essential to reframe the self-image of the community psychiatrist to maintain high self-esteem by reinforcing the notion that this is meaningful and valuable work.
3. The community psychiatrist's role must be managed to maintain variety, interest, and the best use of one's skills and time.
4. It is important to maintain clarity and some sense of personal control over the relationship between the psychiatrist's responsibilities and the authority needed to carry out good clinical care. Sometimes one can develop informal influence that is equivalent to and often not as alienating as authority that is overt and hierarchical.
5. There is a need to remain flexible and to be willing to compromise when necessary. Standards of care have to be balanced at times against the demands for service. This is the most difficult aspect of public psychiatric practice and demands that adequate funding be provided to prevent the erosion of ethical standards.
6. The community psychiatrist must be a creative and innovative leader in the development and use of staff and resources.
7. Attention must be paid to socio-political issues, both global and local, that affect the health and care of patients as well as the health and care of the community mental health program and the larger mental health program within which it functions. The psychiatrist's involvement in social issues can serve as a positive model for both staff and patients.
8. The psychiatrist must understand the system within which he or she works. It is important to know where and how to intervene and to develop the ability to be strategically assertive or tactfully subtle, when necessary, to effect positive changes within the system.

Community mental health program administrators are acutely aware of the shortage of good psychiatrists to work in their programs. The validity of this assertion is supported by the high number of advertisements for psychiatric positions in publications related to community mental health. The following are suggestions of attitudes and behaviors that mental health program administrators can develop in order to be more successful in recruiting and retaining quality community psychiatrists.

1. Offer fair compensation. This should include the option for the psychiatrist to be on contract or salary, depending on his or her preference. Salaried psychiatrists who receive benefits from the agency are more likely to become more visibly integrated members of the program staff.
2. Provide liability insurance. It is important to honor the psychiatrist with at least the same level of liability protection afforded to other staff.
3. Integrate the psychiatrist into the staff so that support for the medical/psychiatric perspective is acknowledged and maintained.
4. Negotiate a flexible and broad variety of functions, including some administrative and teaching functions, if desired by the psychiatrist. The value of the biopsychosocial model can best be demonstrated to the rest of the staff if the psychiatrist's role is not narrowly limited to activities that are superficially deemed most "cost effective."
5. Establish the clear understanding among all staff that the psychiatrist's responsibility is to provide meaningful supervisory input into the care of patients before signing insurance and treatment planning documents.
6. Encourage collaborative approaches to patient care such that when psychiatrists see patients, families, or community groups, other involved clinicians are present as much as possible and as warranted.

There is no question that the world of community mental health has changed dramatically since the early 1960s and 1970s. It is unlikely that there can be a return to the times when psychiatrists were prevalent as administrators or directors. There is also no question that most mental health professionals are highly skilled and dedicated to the provision of high-quality care to their patients. However, the ways that psychiatrists are perceived and utilized in community programs can have a tremendously positive impact on the overall quality of care provided and on the work environment as well. The psychiatrist can and should be a respected partner on the mental health team. Important tasks include providing leadership, modeling clinical skills, imparting knowledge, guiding treatment, listening to and learning from other members of the team, and participating in the overall operation of the center.

David A. Pollack, MD, is Adjunct Associate Professor, Department of Psychiatry, Oregon Health Sciences University, and Medical Director of Mental Health Services West in Portland, Oregon. Dr. Pollack may be contacted at Department of Psychiatry, Oregon Health Sciences University, Portland, OR 97201.

David L. Cutler, MD, is Professor of Psychiatry and Director of the Public Psychiatry Training Program, Department of Psychiatry, Oregon Health Sciences University in Portland, Oregon. He is also the editor of the *Community Mental Health Journal.* Dr. Cutler can be contacted at Department of Psychiatry, Oregon Health Sciences University, Portland, OR 97201.

REFERENCES

Bass, R. D. (1978). *C.M.H.C. Staffing: Who Minds the Store?* Rockville, MD: National Institute of Mental Health.

Caplan, G. (1963). *Principles of Preventive Psychiatry.* New York: Basic Books.

Clark, G. (1988). *Guidelines for Psychiatric Practice in Community Mental Health Settings.* Unpublished document prepared by the Task Force on Professional Practice Issues in Organized Care Settings. Washington, DC: American Psychiatric Association and American Association of Community Psychiatrists.

Clark, G., & Vaccaro, J. (1987). Burnout among CMHC psychiatrists and the struggle to survive. *Hospital and Community Psychiatry, 38,* 843-847.

Cutler, D. L., Bloom, J. D., & Shore, J. H. (1981). Training psychiatrists to work with community support systems for chronically mentally ill persons. *American Journal of Psychiatry, 138,* 98-101.

Dewey, L., & Astrachan, B. M. (1985). Organizational issues in recruitment and retention of psychiatrists by CMHCs. In American Psychiatric Association and National Council of Community Mental Health Centers (Ed.), *Community Mental Health Centers and Psychiatrists* (pp. 22-31). Washington, DC: American Psychiatric Association.

Diamond, H., Cutler, D., Langsley, D., & Barter, J. (1985). Training, recruitment, and retention of psychiatrists in CMHCs: Issues and answers. In American Psychiatric Association and National Council of Community Mental Health Centers (Ed.), *Community Mental Health Centers and Psychiatrists* (pp. 32-50). Washington, DC: American Psychiatric Association.

Engel, G. (1982). The biopsychosocial model in medical education. *New England Journal of Medicine, 306,* 802-805.

Faulkner, L. R., Eaton, J. S., Bloom, J. D., & Cutler, D. L. (1982). The CMHC as a setting for residency education. *Community Mental Health Journal, 18,* 3-10.

Knox, M. D. (1985, September). National register reveals profile of service providers. *National Council News,* p. 1.

Lindemann, E. (1944). Symptomatology and management of acute grief. *American Journal of Psychiatry, 101,* 141-148.

Pardes, H., Pincus, H., & Pomeranz, R. (1985). Foreword. In American Psychiatric Association and National Council of Community Mental Health Centers (Ed.), *Community Mental Health Centers and Psychiatrists* (pp. 1-6). Washington, DC: American Psychiatric Association.

Peterson, L. G. (1981). On being a necessary evil at a mental health center. *Hospital and Community Psychiatry, 32,* 644.

Shore, J. H., Kinzie, D., & Bloom, J. D. (1979). Required educational objectives in community psychiatry. *American Journal of Psychiatry, 136,* 193-195.

Talbott, J. (1979). Why psychiatrists leave the public sector. *Hospital and Community Psychiatry, 30,* 778-782.

Vaccaro, J., & Clark, G. (1987). A profile of community mental health center psychiatrists: Results of a national survey. *Community Mental Health Journal, 23,* 48-55.

7

Community
Mental Health Center
Staff Development
for Service to
Special Populations

David S. Hargrove

Requirements for community mental health centers (CMHCs) to serve special populations create needs for training staff at virtually every level. The special population that has had the greatest impact on community mental health centers in the past 20 years is the long-term seriously mentally ill (Goldman, Regier, & Taube, 1980). Currently, this impact is reinforced by Public Law 99-660, the planning legislation in which the federal government mandates states to develop plans for community-based services for long-term seriously mentally ill persons, homeless long-term seriously mentally ill persons, and children and adolescents.

Community mental health centers have grappled with service delivery to chronically mentally ill (CMI) persons at least since the 1970s, when state government became involved in the funding and administration of programs. Previously, there was a tendency for seriously mentally ill persons to be placed in state psychiatric hospitals. This left community mental health centers to work either with people who were less disturbed or with those who were seriously ill but whose pathologies were in early stages of development. The primary services were short-term care and consultation, education, and prevention programs.

The continued development of community mental health centers, the deinstitutionalization of public psychiatric hospitals, and the state's involvement in the total system of care altered the original mission of community programs. This change reflected the need for service delivery to many of those persons who previously were committed to state facilities.

Such services as precommitment screening, transitional living, rehabilitation, and residential care became commonplace in community programs. Some of the skills needed for working in these programs were different from those needed to provide the original five essential services: short-term inpatient, outpatient, partial hospitalization, 24-hour emergency, and consultation and education. Community centers' new emphasis on services to a more seriously ill clientele identified deficits in the skills of mental health professional, paraprofessional, and nonprofessional staffs. Dealing with a different set of problems brought by persons who were more disturbed for greater periods of time and who had histories of involvement with the mental health system frequently was problematic for community mental health personnel on both the administrative and clinical levels. Unfortunately, little if any empirical study was done to verify whether these changes caused serious problems in service delivery or whether they were deficits associated with attitude or skills, or both, of service providers.

Familiarity with community mental health centers and the growing system through the 1970s revealed, however, some discomfort on the part of providers who were thrown into service delivery with a different kind of client, particularly those characterized by chronicity. Stern and Minkoff (1979) discuss this discomfort in terms of paradoxes in programming for psychiatrists and in training for psychiatric residents (Minkoff & Stern, 1985). It is reasonable to believe that the other core professions - psychology, nursing, and social work - also were equally uncomfortable when faced with different clientele.

Other studies of human resources have shown a lack of preference to work with chronically mentally ill persons across mental health professions. Mirabi et al. (1985) studied mental health professionals in Texas; they found that 85% felt that the chronic mentally ill are not a preferred population with which to work, and 68% thought that most staff persons do not receive adequate training for this work. Moore and M. Davis (1984) found that graduate educators were interested in working with every other client group more than the chronically mentally ill. K. Davis (1987) surveyed 196 graduate students in Virginia to determine their interest in working with chronically mentally ill persons. He found that most were interested in family dysfunction and affective disorders and were only minimally interested in chronic illness.

Staff persons in community mental health programs frequently are faced with clients who demand more than they expect or are trained to handle. The idealism of the young mental health professional can be doused by clients who "expect too much," "respond too little," and have seemingly "insatiable needs." Professionals frequently become less effective and efficient, enjoy their work less, and become vulnerable to professional "burnout." They are likely to seek other employment opportunities, increasing the turnover rate in the public sector. Excessive turnover rates are financially costly and create gaps in the continuity of service delivery to clients.

The purpose of this chapter is to identify the staff development issues resulting from the change in target populations for community mental health programs and to discuss some methods for enabling staff to serve these people and their families more effectively. The first section focuses on preservice training in the previously identified four core professions of psychiatry, psychology, social work, and nursing. Preservice training refers to the basic professional training in a given profession or academic discipline. For example, psychiatrists must complete basic medical training and serve a psychiatric residency prior to their specialization. Clinical psychologists complete an academic PhD program including a clinical internship prior to entering the service delivery sector. Social workers complete a postbaccalaureate MSW degree as preparation for clinical practice. Nurses complete baccalaureate and frequently master's programs in psychiatric nursing before specializing in this field. Specific programs for training professional persons in these fields are identified and discussed. The principle emphasis is on psychology, social work, and nursing; training issues for psychiatrists are covered in Chapter 6 by D. A. Pollack and D. L. Cutler (pp. 125-139).

The second section in this chapter focuses on continuing education for staff who have completed preservice training and have experience in the field. Staff who have worked in community mental health programs include the four core professions but typically expand to embrace a wide variety of professional, paraprofessional, and nonprofessional persons. Community mental health programs have a rich history of involving various types of individuals and professionals in their service programs. Among these are indigenous workers, former clients, and others who are unique to particular communities. This practice has declined as centers rely more on direct payment for services, but some components of public sector mental health continue to rely on staff members who are trained in other perspectives than the four core professions. This section discusses some of the issues of continuing education of community mental health staff and identifies several models for addressing them.

Serving the chronically mentally ill presents unique challenges for professional staff persons in the public sector mental health system. The needs of this population require attention by the total mental health system. This attention is demonstrated by the configuration of the system itself and the skills of the service providers who work within the system.

In order to serve this population effectively, the various components of the system must function in harmony. There needs to be sufficient "continuity of care," not only within one agency, but throughout the entire system. The *National Plan for the Chronically Mentally Ill* (1980) stated:

> Each community, in order to provide for the needs of its citizens who suffer from chronic mental illness, must have the capacity to meet the basic life support needs of these individuals and their treatment (health, mental health), rehabilitative, and social support needs. The community may need to assist the individual in integrating the disparate parts of the system. And the community must recognize and be capable of responding to the fact that the person's needs are often long-term and they both change and fluctuate in intensity over time. (p. 3)

Additionally, the system must be designed to be responsive to the families of chronically ill persons.

Effective service to chronically mentally ill persons within a newly configured system is based on different sets of skills than have been used with other consumers of mental health services. Traditional psychotherapeutic services have not been demonstrated to be effective with chronically mentally ill persons. Combinations of medicine and psychosocial rehabilitation services have been more effective. Providing this mental health care in conjunction with the necessary medical and social services requires different provider skills. Although several models of service delivery have been developed, including Anthony's rehabilitation program at Boston University (Anthony, M. Cohen, & B. Cohen, 1983), Liberman's UCLA program (Liberman &

Phipps, 1987), and Paul and Lentz's system of care (1977), no comprehensive, systematic model of treatment, rehabilitation, and social services has been identified. Consequently, each state and community mental health program is left to forge effective principles of practice with current systems of care.

The few preservice training and continuing education programs that have emerged to meet human resource needs are based on different principles and are designed for different systems of service delivery. Frequently, these systems reflect differences in geographic region, profession and heritage, and philosophies of assessment and intervention. Turf battles and idiosyncratic professionalism can result from these differences unless sufficient communication takes place both *within and across* systems and training programs. Fortunately, the National Institute of Mental Health has sponsored training conferences, and the National Alliance for the Mentally Ill has developed curriculum committees on the national and state levels. These efforts can enhance communication between practitioners and educators and among educators from various professions.

PRESERVICE TRAINING

Preservice training consists of the academic and professional training programs that prepare professional persons for work in the service delivery sector. The typical programs involve baccalaureate levels of education and the specialized training necessary for entry into a profession. Psychiatrists complete premedical and medical training before entering the psychiatric residency. Training to become a clinical psychologist involves undergraduate education, typically in psychology, before entering graduate school, which includes an internship as a part of the PhD program. Social work programs may be at the baccalaureate level but typically follow the undergraduate degree and offer MSW degrees, which include both academic work and practical training. Nursing training is characterized by specialized training to sit for the registered nurse examinations. Baccalaureate, master's, and doctoral degree programs are available in psychiatric nursing. Although there are other relevant training programs for community mental health work, these four professions have been identified as core by the National Institute of Mental Health in early community mental health legislation. Whether they continue to maintain this level of prominence remains to be seen.

145

This discussion will highlight issues of preservice preparation for administration and clinical service delivery in community contexts for work with the chronically mentally ill and their families. The treatment of psychology, social work, and nursing is presented in some detail, leaving the major presentation on psychiatry to Pollack and Cutler (see Chapter 6, pp. 125-139).

PSYCHIATRY

The profession of psychiatry has carried the burden for treating chronically mentally ill persons in the United States at least since the 19th century (Cutler, 1988). Typically this care was provided in state institutions. Cutler and others (Faulkner & Eaton, 1979) point out that although psychiatry was meaningfully involved in the community mental health movement in the United States during its early years, this involvement decreased considerably in the 1980s (Winslow, 1979). In reporting the results of a national survey of psychiatrists, Vaccaro and Clark (1987) indicated that psychiatrists thought they had too much responsibility, insufficient authority, lack of respect from other mental health professionals, and insufficient variety in their jobs. Writing prescriptions became the dominant activity of psychiatrists, and they had little opportunity to supervise staff for whom they were responsible. Additionally, they had no role in the establishment of policy.

Although psychiatrists have been leaving community mental health centers for a variety of reasons, there are forces that require the intense involvement of psychiatrists in community programs. As Peterson (1981) put it, psychiatrists are a "necessary evil" for community mental health centers. Cutler (1988) points out that since the treatment of the chronically mentally ill has become a major focus of community mental health programs, psychiatrists have become invaluable members of CMHC staffs; he claims that "no other discipline is as broadly trained and has as long a tradition in administering to this population" (p. 6). He adds that for psychiatrists to maintain their proper role in service to the chronically mentally ill, "psychiatrists must be trained in some kind of environment that includes the creativity, the value system, and the practical survival skills of the public sector" (p. 6).

Cutler, Bloom, and Shore (1981) have addressed the training of psychiatrists for work with the chronically mentally ill in community mental health contexts. It is significant to note that Cutler, in this and other writings, consistently has advocated the interdisciplinary work of psychiatry and other mental health professions when they are in the community context. This principle underlies many of the efforts to train psychiatrists for public sector work with chronically mentally ill persons.

PSYCHOLOGY

Clinical psychologists are trained in different contexts than psychiatrists, social workers, or nurses. Although these three professions typically train in their own schools with their own deans and some degree of control over their curricula and procedures, psychology departments in most universities are lodged in administrative units that include other diverse disciplines. For example, in most universities, psychology departments are located within colleges of arts and sciences, headed by deans whose base discipline may be any of those in the college. This may include history, English, chemistry, or physics, among a host of others.

The difficulty that this poses for clinical training varies from institution to institution. Typically, the introduction of a professional training program with relatively rigid constraints imposed from outside accrediting agencies as well as ethical guidelines promulgated by nonuniversity sources creates a different context from those whose training is in a school that is essentially controlled by the profession.

The predominant model of training clinical psychologists is the Boulder Model (American Psychological Association, 1949). This model is based on both the scientific and professional roles of the clinical psychologist. Psychologists were to be trained with all academic and methodological rigor as fully qualified psychologists and then as clinicians. Early in its development, clinical training occurred in a Veterans' Administration hospital or similar facility. This model was developed by a study group and adopted by a training conference in Boulder, Colorado, in 1949. It has been reaffirmed in subsequent training conferences.

Presently, however, the development of professional schools of psychology has raised a significant challenge to the predominance of the Boulder training model. Professional schools, granting either the PhD or the PsyD degrees, may focus on professional training for the practice of psychology at the expense of scientific training. Of course, if the programs seek accreditation by the American Psychological Association, there are certain requirements that must be met.

Although psychology has made a significant contribution to the understanding and treatment of chronic mental illness, particularly schizophrenia (Meehl, 1962; Paul & Lentz, 1977; Shakow, 1946), it has been suggested that its unique contribution to the broad field of mental health care is in its empirical methodology (Hersen & Bellack, 1984). Hersen and Bellack point out that one of the essential differences between psychologists and psychiatrists is that psychologists are trained as scientists as well as clinicians. This is the essential point made by Shakow (1947) in the earliest designation of the Boulder model for training clinical psychologists. This dual value maintains a commitment to empirical research to undergird practice.

K. Davis (1987), however, has shown that psychologists have the least interest in practicing where chronically mentally ill persons likely are located - state psychiatric hospitals and Veterans' Administration hospitals. He further pointed out that in his survey of psychology graduate students in Virginia training programs, very few indicated any interest in working with schizophrenic persons.

Psychologists clearly are not on the forefront of service delivery to chronically mentally ill persons. Furthermore, training in psychology appears to be moving in other directions. Unfortunately, there are no guidelines similar to those in psychiatry that provide a criterion for training psychologists for service to chronic mentally ill persons. There are, however, several academic clinical training programs that do train psychologists to work with chronically mentally ill persons (Hargrove & Spaulding, 1988; Johnson, 1988). These programs, located at the University of Nebraska-Lincoln and the University of Houston (Texas), have specialty training for PhD-level students for work with chronically mentally ill persons. Although the programs are somewhat different in structure, they are based on similar values and provide similar training experiences.

There are three major components of a program that seeks to train clinical psychologists for work with the chronically mentally ill. First is the experimental approach to assessment. Because of the discontinuity of assessment and intervention strategy, the functional assessment is an appropriate method of evaluating clients for services. Anthony and his associates at the Boston University rehabilitation program have refined this procedure and provide special training (Anthony & B. Cohen, 1984; Anthony, M. Cohen, & Nemec, 1987).

148

The second major component of clinical psychology training for work with chronically mentally ill persons is in community psychology. Community psychology is an orientation that enables psychologists to work within the larger context in which service delivery systems function. Awareness of collateral agencies, regulatory agencies, legal issues, and the general community in which service delivery takes place is essential for adequate psychological service delivery. This orientation is documented in the growing literature in community psychology, including the account of the National Conference on Training in Community Psychology (Iscoe, B. L. Bloom, & Spielberger, 1977). It also sensitizes psychologists to the needs of families of the chronically mentally ill.

The third major component of clinical psychology training for work with chronically mentally ill persons is in the integration of research and practice. The unique perspective of the Boulder model-trained psychologist is the empirical methodology. This provides an experimental model from which to approach the problems of practicing psychology in public sector agencies with chronically mentally ill persons. Psychologists can thus make a contribution to the clinical care of chronically mentally ill persons as well as to the body of knowledge pertaining to both treatment programs and mental health policy.

Hargrove and Spaulding (1988) have developed a curriculum for a chronic mental illness specialty in clinical psychology that is grounded in these components. Students who commit to this specialty spend practicum placements in both institutional and community settings that serve the chronically mentally ill. They are expected to use their prior research training to address issues of importance to service delivery or administration of services to chronically mentally ill persons. Additionally, they are expected to have at least one course and some practicum experience at the community level. The goal of the specialty is to prepare psychologists who can function in a number of different settings at a number of different levels. For example, these persons are able to serve as clinical service providers or supervisors on a variety of units that provide direct care in both institutional and community settings. They also are prepared to serve in administrative roles, including direct administration of service facilities and in policy and analysis positions at the community, state, or national level.

Although the profession and discipline of psychology has moved in directions away from service to chronically mentally ill persons, there still are a few programs that provide both clinical and research training for persons committed to this population.

These programs provide specialty training for service to chronically mentally ill persons, but many other academic psychology training programs provide generic training based on the values inherent in the scientist-professional model. With appropriate clinical experience, psychologists from these programs are prepared for service to the chronically mentally ill and their families.

SOCIAL WORK

The multiple needs of chronically mentally ill persons and their families demand the presence of social work. Social workers characteristically bring an ecological perspective to service delivery that assures comprehensiveness in the assessment, treatment implementation, and aftercare of the chronically mentally ill.

Rapp and Hanson (1988) have articulated the conclusions from social work research that lay the groundwork for the development of a training curriculum for master's level social workers. The research findings do not mandate a paradigm shift for social work training for service to chronically mentally ill persons. They do establish the parameters for the development of a model curriculum to train social workers for their various roles in service delivery and administration to this population. Paulson (1988) developed a model of social work training that is based on values that are quite similar to those articulated by Rapp and Hanson. He finds that there is no need for a shift from the traditional social work training paradigm.

Rapp and Hanson identify six important conclusions from social work research that inform the development of the curriculum:

1. Psychosocial services with psychotropic medication reduce relapse rates and hospitalization rates and increase community tenure, while psychosocial services with psychotherapy without medication may be harmful.
2. Involvement with families, particularly providing educational materials in a nonblaming manner, brings strongest results in reducing relapse rates.
3. Behavioral and problem-solving strategies are most effective in most settings.
4. Clients know what care and treatment are best for them.

5. Environmental interventions are essential to integrate chronically mentally ill persons into communities.
6. Service delivery outreach enhances client outcomes.

Rapp and Hanson based their three-component curriculum on these findings. The three components consist of practice classes, field practicum, and specialized coursework.

Avoiding the development of special practice classes for services to chronically mentally ill persons, they describe the enrichment of existing practice classes by a two-step process. First, based on current research, they identify missing aspects of existing course offerings. Second, they integrate the content on the chronically mentally ill into the existing classes. Those tasks that are important in the model of adequate service delivery to chronically mentally ill persons are underscored in the courses. Examples of these tasks are the importance of aggressive outreach, partnerships with families, environmental intervention, and the attending to the physiological processes of the illness.

Stressing the importance of field practicum for the training of practitioners, Rapp and Hanson (1988) identify the following characteristics of field placements: (a) experienced supervisors with attitudes consonant with research findings; (b) regular, intensive, and available nonscheduled supervision; (c) case assignment to students early in the placement; and (d) supervisors' focus on observable client outcomes for treatment planning.

The third component of the curriculum consists of special courses. Content of these courses should be in at least two categories: (a) a foundation on which community integration and current treatment approaches may be based, and (b) clinical knowledge necessary for work with the chronically mentally ill. Rapp and Hanson provide the details of these categories, as well as the organizational principles for integrating them into existing social work curricula. Paulson (1988) points out that the integration of classroom activity and field practice is a salient issue, particularly as it affects the knowledge-skill balance in the preparation of professional social workers.

Rapp and Hanson (1988) complete the development of their curriculum with a discussion of management training, which is a part of social work education. This is predicated on the belief that effective service delivery programs must be guided by enlightened, competent management. "Too often quality services are prevented by management which does not provide the necessary direction, the tools, and the rewards" (pp. 11-12). Paulson

(1988), too, believes that social workers trained to work with chronically mentally ill persons must be prepared to be clinical case managers with individual caseloads or to be involved in program administration and policy development.

Many social workers feel that the master's degree is necessary for the most effective practice with the chronically mentally ill. Social workers with the MSW degree have a greater knowledge base and skill development than the BSW practitioners. The possibility of Doctor of Social Work or PhD degrees in social work is raised by Paulson as being relevant to training for service to chronically mentally ill persons. He questions whether the amount of preparation necessary for clinical practice with mentally ill persons is greater than the traditional 2-year social work program. Although there are educators and professionals who argue on both sides of this issue, there appears to be no conclusive answer at this point.

Social work is a crucial profession for effective service delivery to chronically mentally ill persons and their families. The number of social workers in the work force is quite large. Foley (1983) points out that social workers make up the largest group of professionals in the mental health work force. Further, according to Rubin and Gibelman (1984), one of the strongest areas of current social work research is community-based care of the chronically mentally ill.

The ecological perspective and the comprehensive array of tasks that social workers can bring to the clinical and case management situation are invaluable components of the service delivery system. At least in some areas, social work education is maintaining a high profile in training potential staff for work with the chronically mentally ill and their families.

PSYCHIATRIC NURSING

Psychiatric nursing provides a large proportion of the mental health work force. Several sources report that nurses provide more direct patient care hours than any of the mental health professions and that there are more nurses employed in the system than other professions. These data reflect, of course, both inpatient and outpatient services. Fox and Chamberlain (1988) point out that although there are many nurses in the system, it is not completely clear how they contribute to the care of psychiatric patients or the knowledge and competencies necessary for nursing practice. They propose that the heritage of nursing and the influence of psychiatry has led to a focus on the "daily adaptation, function, comfort, health status, and quality of life of individuals, families, and communities" (pp. 1-2).

Traditionally nurses have been prepared to practice at several levels. Prebaccalaureate and baccalaureate-level nurses may become registered nurses and enter the field of practice at those levels. Persons with these qualifications practice within a generalist mode. A nurse with a bachelor's degree in nursing may have beginning skills in psychiatric nursing.

Further academic and clinical preparation can lead to a master's degree with a specialization, including psychiatry. Fox and Chamberlain (1988) point out, "This specialization is directed specifically toward the development of advanced clinical skills in psychiatric nursing practice and requires the acquisition of knowledge about psychopathology and psychopharmacology" (p. 298). Students must develop specific skills through academic and clinical supervision. "For instance," they point out, "a master's nursing student in psychiatric nursing with a subspecialty in chronic mental illness would be required to have advanced preparation in skills and knowledge related to chronicity, community support, and psychosocial rehabilitation" (p. 3). The master's nurse is considered to be an advanced practitioner.

Although doctoral programs in nursing are developing, their primary contribution is to the development of scientists who conduct research in applied nursing care.

Although attention to training mental health professionals for work with the chronically mentally ill has been lacking, a few training programs have been developed in each of the core mental health professions. Additionally, advocacy groups have become involved in training issues and can provide assistance and consultation to training programs seeking to develop programs. The National Alliance for the Mentally Ill, for example, has developed a training committee and has held at least one national conference on training professional persons.

CONTINUING EDUCATION

The intent of the initial federal community mental health legislation was to serve the mental health needs of the entire community. These needs had both direct and indirect components of service. Direct services included inpatient, outpatient, partial hospitalization, and emergency service components. Indirect services included consultation and education, or prevention services. Public Law 94-63 both expanded the services and specified target populations for community mental health programs.

In 1981, categorical granting programs were phased out in favor of block grants. Block grants are single amounts of money given to states for purposes consistent with mental health plans. This funding mechanism allowed the shift of priorities from the national level to the state level. The emphasis on serving the chronically mentally ill, already begun in the mid 1970s, was strengthened. Jerrell and Larsen (1986) reported a shift in funding patterns of community mental health centers as a result of the block grant system. Their data showed that services to chronically mentally ill persons and severely acutely mentally ill persons received more support from states.

This emphasis on chronically mentally ill persons was a shift from the broader perspective of the target populations in the initial mandate. Although it made a substantial difference in mental health policy at the national and state levels, it made an equally substantial difference in the local community mental health center. The difference was found in the day-to-day work of clinical staff persons who delivered the services. Persons who previously were considered candidates for institutionalization were hospitalized for a brief period and returned to the community, where treatment and support were expected. Persons who had been institutionalized for longer periods were released to the communities for treatment and care in the "least restrictive alternative."

These new clients brought new needs that dictated changes in the skills required of effective staff members. It was not particularly useful for staff persons to use the traditional methods of psychotherapy with chronically mentally ill persons, who were in desperate need of a stable environment, medication, housing, and training for personal and social skills. In fact, Drake and Sederer (1986) show that intensive psychotherapy has potentially negative effects on people suffering from schizophrenia. Although a variety of programs have emerged to serve chronically mentally ill persons in communities, there is little evidence to suggest that community mental health center staffs have adopted different treatment modalities for the CMI population for which they are responsible. Johnson (1989) writes:

Therapies intended to resolve experience-based conflicts (e.g., the insight-oriented, dynamic psychotherapies) should be reserved for different groups of clients, those for whom brain dysfunction is not an issue, and should not be used with seriously mentally ill individuals. At present, however, these forms of psychotherapy are still being used in community mental health centers, hospitals, and private offices throughout the country, at great expense to patients, relatives, and the public and despite the absence of empirical evidence of effectiveness. (p. 554)

Providing services that are relevant and useful to chronically mentally ill persons and families requires different skills from those needed in the early years of community mental health centers.

From a different perspective, Lefley and Cutler (1988) suggest that there never has been specific training of human resources to provide the services that community mental health centers made available, particularly in the context of deinstitutionalization:

The [community mental health center] movement began with great expectations that somehow severely mentally ill people could be removed from hospitals and treated in the new community mental health centers. However, no one prepared the mental health centers for what they were supposed to be doing and no one prepared the staff of those centers with skill, attitude, and knowledge bases that fit the needs of the target population. (p. 253)

It has been demonstrated that training professional mental health resources for work with the chronically mentally ill has been quite slow in developing (Anthony, M. Cohen, & Farkas, 1988; Lefley & Cutler, 1988). Further, as the community mental health system changed to emphasize service delivery to the chronically mentally ill, systematic continuing education programs have not emerged to equip existing staff for their new responsibilities. The expected result of this state of affairs, quite reasonably, is that people continue to do what they were trained to do. Because neither professional training programs nor continuing education offerings have addressed these needs, mental health staff persons do not have the opportunity to develop the necessary skills.

There are other reasons for the lack of opportunities for skill development in service delivery to chronically mentally ill persons. The nature of the development of the community mental health system in the various states varies considerably. With that variation in development are the differences in the structures of the state systems. For example, the relationships among the state mental health authority, the state institutions, and the community mental health centers vary. Additionally, the relationships between the state authority, hospitals, and centers and colleges and universities differ from state to state and even within individual states.

Another set of issues that influence the development of skills following professional training is lodged in the individual professions that are represented in the public sector. Psychiatry, psychology, social work, and nursing, as well as other professions involved in mental health practice, have different rules and expectations for continuing education. Each of the professions is quite different in the development of continuing education requirements for its members. The requirements usually are determined by individual state licensure agencies and professional groups. For example, state boards in different states that regulate the practice of psychology vary in whether continuing education is required for ongoing licensure. The relationship between the various professional groups, particularly in continuing education, remains largely unexplored.

An important concern of continuing education is the determination of the skills or knowledge that is to be developed. The changes in the public sector of mental health service delivery include the constituencies who have vital interests in the types of skills that mental health providers possess. These constituencies include persons who are involved in governance, service delivery, and administration; consumers; and family members of consumers. A number of organizations represent these groups of people. One example is the National Alliance for the Mentally Ill, which has become heavily involved in promoting research and training for work with seriously mentally ill persons. Each of these constituency groups represents a perspective of service delivery and can assist in developing a comprehensive understanding of the skills needed by mental health staff persons to work in public sector service delivery.

Silverman (1980, 1981) has designed continuing education programs for several levels of community mental health staff members. Using his perspective as a community psychologist, he sought extensive input from all the persons involved in continuing education to determine the content and format of the programs.

Since Silverman's work in Illinois, the constituencies of the mental health service delivery system have crystallized and articulated their values. A program of continuing education that would meet the needs of the modern community mental health center should follow Silverman's model of community support to receive direct input from its constituency groups. This model would insure that persons in governance, administrators, supervisory and line staff, interested representatives of consumer and family groups, and other concerned groups in the community would be directly involved in the articulation of the skills and knowledge necessary for adequate service delivery.

The use of a broad base of constituencies in a community for shaping staff training can lead to a significant opportunity for communication between the various components of the mental health system. This communication has the potential for greater involvement of these groups in the total program of the community mental health program, which enhances its capability for effective service delivery.

Both professional training in mental health and continuing education for existing staff persons have been slow to address the specific target populations that community mental health centers must address. Several reasons for this have been provided. The solution to the problem appears to lie in the value of the *community* basis of the community mental health center. The contribution of the community's components that are relevant to mental health service delivery can both enhance the training efforts of the program and lead to other powerful relationships.

IMPLEMENTING STAFF
DEVELOPMENT PROGRAMS

Community mental health centers have changed considerably since their inception in the early 1960s (Woy, Wasserman, & Weiner-Pomerantz, 1981). Even with the variation between states in their administration of the programs, CMHC budgets generally have become tighter and less flexible. Programs that do not yield direct revenue are in danger of being eliminated. This belt-tightening has forced administrators to reconsider the importance of staff development, probably because of a lack of data to demonstrate effectiveness as well as reduced budgets. As continuing training opportunities are less available to staff, a serious danger of staff stagnation emerges to threaten the quality of care provided by the agency. This danger, along with the newly interpreted needs and recommended services to the major client population of agencies in the public sector, creates a dilemma for workers in these agencies.

This section sets forth a systematic procedure for the identification of staff needs for service to chronically mentally ill persons. This procedure is followed by a description of an assessment of resources to meet those needs and suggestions for implementation and evaluation of staff development activities. The procedures are designed for centers with varying resources. The purpose is to maintain the principles of accountability to governing bodies, the community that supports the agency, and consumers. It is hoped that they represent the same spirit of accountability that is contained in the original community mental health center's legislation.

It is important to point out that "skills" are only one component of what is needed for effective work with the chronically mentally ill. Minkoff (1987), citing Neilson et al. (1982), noted that the interplay of knowledge, skills, and attitudes with adequate supervision and appropriate role models characterize successful training programs. The development of knowledge and attitudes conducive to serving the chronically mentally ill must accompany skill acquisition for service delivery to be effective. Thus, knowledge, skills, and attitudes are appropriate topics for staff development. In the subsequent discussion, the term "skills" is used to represent knowledge and attitudes as well.

NEEDS/RESOURCE ASSESSMENT

The needs assessment for staff development must reflect the various constituencies of the mental health agency. These constituencies with their various interests represent often diverse perspectives that influence mental health service agencies. It is important that these perspectives influence the training and skill development of all levels of staff in the agency. The combination of influences assures that staff are prepared to deliver meaningful and relevant services and that the constituency groups share a sense of ownership of the agency.

In most community mental health agencies there are at least six overlapping constituency groups that should influence the agency, including the values that shape the training of staff. They include (a) the community in its broadest concept, (b) the consumers of the agency, (c) the board of directors charged with governance of the agency, (d) the administration employed by the

158

board, (e) the staff that provide the services, and (f) the agency's funding sources.

The community at large is the broadest constituency that influences the agency. The values that it affirms will shape the mission and programs of the facility through the formal and informal governance structures. The community-as-constituency is accessed through its traditional governmental, political, and social structures that have official relationships to public sector mental health agencies, for example, county and city governing boards, advisory groups to the agency, and other structures that may be unique to specific local programs. It is also important that the community-as-constituency be accessed through nontraditional means to empower individuals and groups who either do not have specific representation through official channels or have interests specific to the mental health agency.

Consumers, a distinct subset of the community, wield a powerful influence on the nature of the services offered. Consumers who directly benefit from services have organized in many communities and are developing effective ways of making their needs known. Additionally, the families of consumers have effective organizations to articulate their needs.

The board of directors of the agency has a direct impact on the mission of the agency by the development and maintenance of policy that reflects the values of the community and the positive practice of mental health service delivery. Administrators frequently are responsible for the interpretation between staff, community, and boards to assure a balanced and accurate perspective.

The administration of the agency presents a different perspective of the necessary services and the skills needed to effectively provide those services. Having specific knowledge of the services required by specific funding sources, for example, puts administrators in a particularly influential position. Also, they are positioned between various constituency groups and direct service providers and frequently must interpret between them. Additionally, administrators typically have their own values that influence service delivery, thus affecting the staff development procedures.

Staff persons who must deliver direct services have the greatest knowledge of being in the helping role with specific populations and must influence the form of service delivery. Also, specific staff members have knowledge of their own strengths and weaknesses in clinical service delivery. Thus, staff persons should have major input in the identification of skills for service delivery and in the process by which they are developed.

Most funding sources have standard-setting responsibilities that influence the services that are provided. These sources include the state departments of mental health, federal agencies that underwrite service delivery programs, or local funding sources that provide funding for mental health care. Typically the United Way or some other organization that coordinates charitable efforts in a community is an example of a local source that might influence the type of services that are provided. The plethora of funding sources that provide support for community programs frequently make responding a complex and often confusing task.

These constituency groups have powerful interests in the services provided by the local agency and thus need access to the policies and procedures of skill development of the staff. They are of course coordinated by the administration of the agency, which mediates conflicting demands for services and skills. In most agencies, the administration of the agency is responsible for establishing the structure in which staff development is implemented. That responsibility makes it imperative that administrators gain perspectives beyond their own for the continuing education of themselves and the staff.

The formulation of a plan for staff development involves at least five steps. They include (a) the articulation of the agency's mission, particularly in relation to a given service program; (b) the definition of service outcomes; (c) the determination of required skills for delivery of the service outcomes; (d) the determination of existing staff skills; and (e) the identification of skill deficits. The difference between existing skills and required skills constitutes the skill deficits. Likewise, differences between existing knowledge or attitudes and required knowledge or attitudes constitute deficits. These deficits provide the basis on which training endeavors may be focused.

The agency's mission typically is determined by the board of directors in response to its interpretation of community needs and legislative mandates from state and county governments. This mission provides the guidance for agency policy and the services that it maintains. Specific outcomes are identified for the services provided. Administrators and service staff determine the skills needed to assure the outcomes of the services and compare these to the skill levels of the existing staff. This comparison results in the deficits, or needs. The knowledge, skills, and attitudes that are needed for effective service delivery provide the focus for training existing staff and hiring new staff to provide the services.

The products of such an assessment include a multilevel definition of the needs of the total staff and an individualized definition of needs for each staff member. The multilevel assessment of the total staff, including every person involved with a particular service, is necessary for differential training programs designed to include everyone involved. For example, it is just as important for the receptionist in a mental health center to know how to relate to a chronically mentally ill person as it is for a psychologist or social worker to know how to treat him or her. The business office of the mental health center must be aware of the mechanisms for payment and the strategies for collection from public and private sources for services to chronically mentally ill persons.

Additionally, an individualized training plan can be developed for each staff member who must work in a specific service. This plan results from the comparison of the current level of functioning with that required by that person's specific responsibilities in the new service. This highly specific, objective approach enables each staff person to develop objectives for his or her own training needs in a given time period. Agreement on these objectives between this staff member and his or her supervisor can constitute a training plan that is specific to the service and to the staff person expected to work in that service.

Just as the agency's and individual staff members' needs must be assessed, the available resources for meeting these needs must be identified. The systematic assessment of resources in a given community inevitably yields unexpected opportunities for the development of knowledge, attitudes, and skills relevant to service delivery. Parenthetically, the utilization of other agencies, professionals, and institutions can enhance the quality of relationships needed in the overall service delivery system. Needed skills that may not be developed with local personnel are identified and assistance can be sought from other resources. For example, if case management skills are needed and resources cannot be found locally, multicounty and state sources may be tapped for the appropriate leadership.

In identifying the resources available in a community, an agency can access the same constituency groups from which perspectives of needs were obtained. Community-at-large, consumer, board, administrative, and staff perspectives should be sought to determine where resources for training and enlightenment may be found.

An investigation of the community-at-large, for example, may yield specific skills and perspectives for working with chronic populations. A reasonable example in many communities is the department of social services or social welfare. Social workers staffing these agencies have been working in services resembling what mental health professionals are calling "case management" for many years. Although the dimensions are not exactly the same, the counsel of welfare social workers may be invaluable to mental health professionals who seek to provide more than the basic mental health services to chronically mentally ill persons. The knowledge of pitfalls, additional resources, and specific persons in the community who may be helpful provide assets to the mental health professionals who provide case management services. Additionally, the working relationship between the welfare department and the community mental health center is enhanced by the CMHC's request for training.

A survey of community resources would include other agencies providing human services, schools and colleges, business and industry, and other facilities unique to specific communities. For example, mental retardation facilities have done case management for years, albeit under a different name. Although case management for persons with chronic mental illness is not identical to that which is done for persons who are retarded, there likely is sufficient overlap to suggest collaboration in staff training.

When the survey of community resources does not yield adequate resources to meet the needs of the mental health center staff, assistance from multiple county groups (districts, regions, or associations developed solely for training purposes) or the state authority should be sought. Associations of centers and the state authority frequently can provide direct assistance or have knowledge of available resources to meet training needs. Lauffer (1977) suggests that continuing education programs can be packaged and exchanged to expand the latitude of their use. He gives a few examples:

> In a midwestern community, three mental health agencies that had conducted successful training programs on three separate topics agreed to swap their programs. The exchange was so successful that they decided to plan future offerings jointly. Each continued to take major responsi-

bility for a particular training topic, but the selection of topics and resource persons was determined jointly. Several professional schools in different parts of the country have engaged in similar enterprises. A successful three-day institute on sociobehavioral techniques conducted by one school was swapped with several other continuing education programs in return for two- or three-day workshops on topics for which the other cooperating institutions were well known. (p. 100)

The product of such a resource survey can be a document in which the resources are matched with the stated needs of multiple levels of staff. From this document, individual training plans can be developed for all staff persons involved in a given service.

CHARACTERISTICS OF TRAINING

There are several characteristics of staff development programs that are important for successful training. These characteristics have to do with the relevance, format, and consistency of the training programs.

The clear relevance of the training to the staff providing the needed services is essential for successful staff development to occur. This relevance should be built in with the procedure for determining the needs that are being addressed. Needs are defined as the differences between existing skills and those which are necessary for providing a service. Staff members, particularly professional persons, may be helped to see that a new service requires new skills by service providers and that it is not realistic to expect that they already should have them. Training, like psychotherapy, progresses more smoothly when the recipients acknowledge the need for it.

One characteristic of relevant training is that it not only be skill development but that it also include training for decision making. It must include both attitudes and knowledge to accompany relevant skills. Asking professional persons simply to apply a skill or a technique to a given population is underutilizing the professional resources and likely oversimplifies the needs of the clientele. Training for decision making is much more relevant to the proper use of professional human resources and enables them to be of considerably more value to the client.

The format of staff development is essential to the receptivity of staff members for the training. It is entirely reasonable that persons who have delivered mental health services for some time will need a different style of training than a new graduate student who has just completed an undergraduate degree. Theoretical foundations should already be in place. Shifts in theoretical orientations are handled quite differently from the development of those orientations.

The technology of adult education, particularly that which is focused on professional development, has grown enormously as the arena for professional activity has expanded in recent years (Lauffer, 1977, 1978; Lenz, 1980; Shortell, 1978). The use of role play, simulation, and case formulations have become effective means of training clinical staff persons to be responsive to their clientele.

Finally, the consistency of training is critical. The training programs should be consistent with the service models that are being followed in the agency. Inconsistency results in confusion of staff and arbitrary choices for future training endeavors. When a service model is developed and its components identified, the training program must relate directly to those components. It does little good to train staff in a clubhouse model of working with persons with chronic mental illness when the actual program is a structured psychosocial rehabilitation program devoted to specific skill development.

Implementation of staff development programs based on the needs and resource assessment depends largely on the magnitude of the agency, the numbers of staff persons affected, and the complexity of the objectives to be attained. The budgets for staff development programs also can range from inexpensive to quite expensive. It is reasonable to believe that the expenses in time, energy, and money will be smaller if the agency's and the individual staff members' training priorities are established and demonstrated to be relevant to the tasks of employment.

It is, of course, essential that agencies plan staff development programs in similar ways that they plan service delivery programs. Objectives for both groups and individuals are identified, strategies for reaching those objectives are developed, resources are identified and deployed, and the practicalities of program management are delegated to the appropriate staff. Evaluation of staff development efforts should focus on the acquisition of skills, knowledge, and attitudes that are relevant to the service outcomes that have been identified. Relevant technologies for the implementation and evaluation of programs are available elsewhere, for example, in Glaser and Kirkhart (1983) and in R. E. Gordon and K. K. Gordon (1980).

CONCLUSION

Clearly, there are several dimensions to the development of the human resources necessary to implement a community mental health system. First, preservice training is essential to prepare professional and nonprofessional workers for their responsibilities in a community level of care. Second, the continued training of both professionals and nonprofessionals is essential to enable these people to maintain their skills and develop new skills to serve changing populations. This chapter has sought to identify some of the issues of human resource development at the community mental health center level. Further, it has sought to provide suggestions for effective human resource planning and staff development for community mental health centers with both great or few resources.

David S. Hargrove, PhD, is currently Professor and Chair of the Department of Psychology at the University of Mississippi in University, Mississippi. He was formerly Director of Human Resource Development for the Virginia Department of Mental Health, Mental Retardation, and Substance Abuse Services, and has served as an Executive Director of a community mental health center. Dr. Hargrove may be contacted at Department of Psychology, University of Mississippi, University, MS 38677.

REFERENCES

American Psychological Association. (1949). Recommended graduate training programs in clinical psychology. *American Psychologist, 2,* 539-558.

Anthony, W., & Cohen, B. (1984). Functional assessment in psychiatric rehabilitation. In A. Halpern & M. Fuhrer (Eds.),

Functional Assessment in Rehabilitation (pp. 79-100). Baltimore: Brookes.

Anthony, W., Cohen, M., & Cohen, B. (1983). The philosophy, treatment process and principles of the psychiatric rehabilitation approach. *New Directions in Mental Health, 17*, 67-79.

Anthony, W., Cohen, M., & Farkas, M. (1988). Professional preservice training for working with the long-term mentally ill. *Community Mental Health Journal, 24*, 258-269.

Anthony, W. A., Cohen, M., & Nemec, P. B. (1987). Assessment in psychiatric rehabilitation. In B. Bolton (Ed.), *Handbook of Measurement and Evaluation in Rehabilitation* (pp. 299-312). Baltimore: Paul Brooks.

Cutler, D. (1988, September). *Training Psychiatric Residents to Work with the Chronically Mentally Ill*. Paper presented at The National Forum for Educating Professionals to Work with the Chronically Mentally Ill, Chevy Chase, MD.

Cutler, D., Bloom, J., & Shore, J. (1981). Training psychiatrists to work in community support systems for chronically mentally ill persons. *American Journal of Psychiatry, 138*, 98-101.

Davis, K. (1987). *The Challenge to State Mental Health Systems and Universities in Virginia: Preparation of Mental Health Professionals for Work with the Chronic Mentally Disabled* (Final Report). Richmond, VA: The Galt Visiting Scholar Chair in Public Mental Health, Commonwealth of Virginia.

Drake, R. E., & Sederer, L. I. (1986). The adverse effects of intensive treatment of chronic schizophrenia. *Comprehensive Psychiatry, 27*, 313-326.

Faulkner, L., & Eaton, J. (1979). Administrative relationships between community mental health centers and academic psychiatric departments. *American Journal of Psychiatry, 196*, 129-136.

Foley, H. (1983). *Madness and Government: Who Cares for the Mentally Ill?* Washington, DC: American Psychiatric Press.

Fox, J., & Chamberlain, J. (1988). Preparing nurses to work with the chronically mentally ill. *Community Mental Health Journal, 24*, 296-309.

Glaser, E. M., & Kirkhart, K. E. (Eds.). (1983). *Cornerstones of Performance: Improving Evaluation in Mental Health Systems*. Austin and Los Angeles: Human Interaction Research Institute.

Goldman, H., Regier, D., & Taube, C. (1980). Community mental health centers and the treatment of severe mental disorder. *American Journal of Psychiatry, 137*, 83-86.

Gordon, R. E., & Gordon, K. K. (1980). *Systems of Treatment for the Mentally Ill: Filling the Gaps*. New York: Grune & Stratton.

Hargrove, D., & Spaulding, W. (1988). Training psychologists for work with the chronically mentally ill. *Community Mental Health Journal, 24*, 283-295.

Hersen, M., & Bellack, A. (1984). Research in clinical psychology. In A. Bellack & M. Hersen (Eds.), *Research Methods in Clinical Psychology* (p. 1). New York: Pergamon.

Iscoe, I., Bloom, B. L., & Spielberger, C. D. (1977). *Community Psychology in Transition*. New York: Wiley.

Jerrell, J. M., & Larsen, J. K. (1986). Community mental health services in transition. *American Journal of Orthopsychiatry, 56*, 78-88.

Johnson, D. L. (1988). Response to "key issues for training in psychology for service to the seriously mentally ill. In H. Lefley (Ed.), *Clinical Training in Serious Mental Illness* (DHHS Publication No. ADM-90-1679). Washington, DC: U.S. Government Printing Office, NIMH, Supt. of Documents.

Johnson, D. L. (1989). Schizophrenia as a brain disease: Implications for psychologists and families. *American Psychologist, 44*, 553-555.

Lauffer, A. (1977). *The Practice of Continuing Education in the Human Services*. New York: McGraw-Hill.

Lauffer, A. (1978). *Doing Continuing Education and Staff Development*. New York: McGraw-Hill.

Lefley, H., & Cutler, D. (1988). Training professionals to work with the chronically mentally ill. *Community Mental Health Journal, 24*, 253-257.

Lenz, E. (1980). *Creating and Marketing Programs in Continuing Education*. New York: McGraw-Hill.

Liberman, R. P., & Phipps, C. C. (1987). Innovative techniques for the chronic mental patient. In W. W. Menninger & G. Hannah, *The Chronic Mental Patient/II*. Washington, DC: American Psychiatric Press.

Meehl, P. (1962). Schizotaxia, schizotypy, schizophrenia. *American Psychologist, 17*, 827-838.

Minkoff, K. (1987). Resistance of mental health professionals to working with the chronic mentally ill. In A. T. Meyerson (Ed.), *Barriers to Treating the Chronic Mentally Ill* (pp. 3-20). San Francisco: Jossey-Bass.

Minkoff, K., & Stern, R. (1985). Paradoxes faced by residents being trained in the psychosocial treatment of people with chronic schizophrenia. *Hospital and Community Psychiatry, 36,* 859-864.

Mirabi, M., Weinman, M., Magnetti, S., & Keppler, K. (1985). Professionals' attitudes toward the chronic mentally ill. *Hospital and Community Psychiatry, 36,* 404-405.

Moore, J., & Davis, M. (1984). *Staff Recruitment and Retention in Community Support Programs: A Ten State Study.* Boulder, Co: Western Interstate Commission for Higher Education.

National Plan for the Chronically Mentally Ill: Report to the Secretary (Final Draft). (1980). Washington, DC: U.S. Department of Health and Human Services.

Neilson, A. C., Stein, L. I., Talbott, J. A., Lamb, H. R., Osser, D. N., & Glazer, W. M. (1982). Encouraging psychiatrists to work with chronic patients: Opportunities and limitations of residency education. *Hospital and Community Psychiatry, 32,* 767-775.

Paul, G., & Lentz, R. (1977). *Psychosocial Treatment of Chronic Mental Patients.* Cambridge, MA: Harvard.

Paulson, R. (1988). Educating social workers to work with long-term seriously mentally ill persons and their families. In H. Lefley (Ed.), *Clinical Training in Serious Mental Illness* (DHHS Publication No. ADM-90-1679). Washington, DC: U.S. Government Printing Office, NIMH, Supt. of Documents.

Peterson, L. (1981). On being a necessary evil at a mental health center. *Hospital and Community Psychiatry, 32,* 664.

Rapp, C. A., & Hanson, J. (1988). Towards a model social work curriculum for practice with the chronically mentally ill. *Community Mental Health Journal, 24,* 270-281.

Rubin, A., & Gibelman, M. (1984). *Social Work Research in Mental Health: The State of the Art.* Rockville, MD: National Institute of Mental Health.

Shakow, D. (1946). The nature of deterioration in schizophrenic condition. *Nervous and Mental Disorders Monograph Series No. 70.* New York: Coolidge Foundation.

Shakow, D. (1947). Recommended graduate training program in clinical psychology. *American Psychologist, 2,* 539-558.

Shortell, S. M. (1978). *Health Program Evaluation.* St. Louis: Mosby.

Silverman, W. H. (1980). Self-designed continuing education for supervisors in community mental health. *Journal of Community Psychology, 9,* 347-354.

Silverman, W. H. (1981). Trainee-designed continuing education in community mental health. *Professional Psychology, 11,* 24-30.

Stern, R., & Minkoff, K. (1979). Paradoxes in programming for chronic patients in a community clinic. *Hospital and Community Psychiatry, 30,* 613-617.

Vaccaro, J. V., & Clark, G. H. (1987). A profile of community mental health center psychiatrists: Results of a national survey. *Community Mental Health Journal, 23,* 282-289.

Winslow, W. (1979). The changing role of psychiatrists in CMHCs. *American Journal of Psychiatry, 136,* 24-27.

Woy, J. R., Wasserman, D. B., & Weiner-Pomerantz, R. (1981). Community mental health centers: Movement away from the model. *Community Mental Health Journal, 4,* 265-276.

Basic Principles in Board Development and Training

James O. Gibson

The role and function of community mental health center governing boards have been discussed since the beginning of the community mental health center movement. What are board members supposed to do? What is the division of responsibility between the board and the executive? Who decides what the respective roles will be? What happens when there is disagreement? How is the information about roles to be communicated?

An abundance of information exists to answer these questions and provide adequate training about board governance for both board members and executives. Yet, the role and function of boards continue to be problematic for many community mental health centers.

Thousands of people in communities throughout the United States serve on boards of community mental health centers. People volunteer personal time to serve on boards, without compensation, in hopes of making a contribution to their communities. The volunteers are usually concerned, committed citizens who care about their communities.

Boards are charged with the responsibility of making significant decisions about the delivery of mental health services within their communities. Because they are composed of people who are representative of the community, governing boards are strategically positioned to influence critical issues regarding the future of community mental health.

A community mental health center board that governs proficiently is a powerful source of strength and support for a center, a chief executive officer, and the staff. A competent governing board provides leadership in major policy issues confronting the center, generates vibrant community support, empowers its executive to manage, and monitors community benefit of center operations.

Board training is fundamental to a successful center. Knowledgeable leadership at the board level is as essential as trained professionals at the clinical level. Today, community mental health centers are facing their greatest challenges. The future of community mental health will depend on the ability of boards to play a major leadership and strategic role in the governance of their respective agencies.

Because the governing board's role is preeminent, the training and development of board members must be given high priority. In most mental health centers, board training is seriously neglected. Some board members have not been provided the basic information required to help them effectively discharge their responsibilities.

Community mental health centers have minimum standards for staff prior to hiring and often require or provide continuing education and training. Yet the training of board members is frequently overlooked. This neglect is a major disservice to the center, the community, and board members themselves. Although they are most likely to be the first victim of an untrained board, executives often focus greater attention on other administrative issues.

RESULTS OF
INADEQUATE BOARD TRAINING

Untrained board members will adapt in one of two ways. First, they will be reluctant to assume leadership for fear of doing something inappropriate. They will attend meetings but usually defer to the executive director on most issues. They may continue on the board, or they may eventually lose interest and resign. A board that fails to provide leadership in governance forfeits to the executive major decisions without board guidance, placing the executive in an extremely vulnerable position if his or her decisions or recommendations have a negative outcome.

Second, board members who are unclear about their role will take an active role and begin to look for something important to do. They may focus on familiar or comfortable issues that are unrelated to their roles as board members. Examples are intrusion into financial management, personnel management, or service delivery matters. They frequently create extensive problems for the center and its chief executive officer by interfering in activity totally inappropriate for boards. A board that makes misguided attempts to play a significant role in the daily operations of the center risks serious and destructive conflict with the executive.

Allowing board members to remain untrained is counterproductive, inexcusable, and unfair to board members who are attempting to provide a valuable service. The situation can lead to internal conflict, inhibit the center's growth, demoralize staff, weaken service delivery, and betray community trust. Such problems can be avoided with an ongoing board development program. A progressive community mental health center director must give special attention to the training of the governing board. The executive must commit both time and money to establish or strengthen a board development program.

INFORMAL BOARD TRAINING

Board training should be a continuous process that promotes interaction of the executive and board members. Every board meeting, every report, and every conversation provides an opportunity to offer informal training for board members. The chief executive officer is the primary trainer of the board - a role model for daily demonstration of the distinctions between the executive role and the governance role. The chief executive officer must understand the governance role in order to nourish and bolster appropriate behaviors. If the executive lacks clarity about board governance, inappropriate behavior of board members is likely to be reinforced.

TRAINING DURING BOARD MEETINGS

The regular board meeting furnishes an excellent forum for the executive to provide informal training for the board. Every action of the executive should be carefully calculated to convey the message of role appropriateness. If the executive takes a position that usurps a role that rightfully belongs to the board, the executive is contributing to role confusion. If the executive asks a question of the board that is a legitimate management issue, the board may intrude in management affairs.

An effective executive will use the following mechanisms during regular board meetings for informal board training.

Board Reports. Reports tend to dominate the discussions that take place at board meetings. Board members will feel compelled to ask questions and make decisions about the information that they receive. If the reports contain management issues, the board will tend to discuss management issues and make management decisions. If the reports contain policy issues, the board will tend to discuss policy issues and make policy decisions.

Reports (both oral and written) provide the executive with an opportunity to help the board focus on appropriate issues. All reports that are presented to the board should contain only information that is needed by the board for governance. Specific informational items that relate to the management of the center need not be included in board reports.

All financial reports, program reports, and administrative reports should be carefully prepared to provide the board with information that will direct its discussions to governance issues that have long-range impact on the organization. The reports should enable the board to focus on decisions that guide the center's future and govern its operation.

Issues Introduced. Issues are introduced in board meetings through both formal and informal methods. Formal methods include reports, presentations, and motions. Informal methods can include almost anything from a direct question to a casual comment by a board member.

The executive must be alert to issues that are raised that distract the board from its governance focus. Often the executive can successfully intervene by referring to an existing policy that governs the issue, diverting the discussion from a narrow focus to broader policy implications, or suggesting that it be referred to committee for study of policy implications. In some situations, the executive may simply explain to the board that the issue is not a governance issue and does not warrant board consideration. The chief executive officer must use considerable tact and skill and find subtle ways to use each issue introduced to help the board better understand its governance role.

Recommendations. Executives must be cautious about making recommendations to the board on policy issues. An executive recommendation can put the board in the position of considering the recommendation rather than the policy issue underlying the recommendation, and put the executive in the position of appearing to supplant the board's policy-making role. Executives are usually sensitive to attempts by boards to interfere in management issues, but they can sometimes unknowingly impinge upon the board's policy-making role by the exertion of undue influence.

The introduction of policy issues to the board or a committee affords the executive an excellent board-training opportunity. By assuming a staff role (information provider, advisor) and allowing the board to assume a board role (policy decision maker), the executive helps the board clearly understand the difference between the board and staff roles.

TRAINING THROUGH PERSONAL INTERACTION

Informal interaction with board members allows the executive to use personal relationship as a training technique. Sitting with the chairperson of the board or a committee to plan a meeting agenda provides an excellent opportunity for focusing the lay leader on policy issues. Individual meetings with board members who may be struggling with role clarification issues or having difficulty chairing a committee provide training opportunities. The skillful executive will be cognizant of the training needs of each board member and search for methods to assist in their training.

TRAINING DURING RECRUITMENT

Most community mental health centers attempt to recruit board members who are already busy people with heavy responsibilities and limited available time. Executives often mistakenly assume that potential board members must be seduced into accepting board membership by minimizing the requirements and responsibilities of the role. Some centers deliberately understate what is expected of board members in order to entice them to serve on the board. This practice is a serious error. Recruitment of people for the board who understand the obligations and expectations of the office and who willingly accept the burdens and limitations of the role is especially important.

Begin the training of board members before they come on to the board. The recruitment process often is the ideal time to educate potential board members about their role and function.

An effective technique is to prepare an inexpensive brochure especially for prospective board members. If cost is an issue, the brochure can be prepared on a typewriter or word processor. The brochure should convey enough information to enable the potential board member to understand the essentials of board governance.

Key topics to be covered in the brochure are:

1. Information about the organization, its services, its financial condition, its organizational structure, and the board.
2. What is expected of board members, including their roles, responsibilities, functions, and duties.
3. The role of the chief executive officer, including duties, relationship to staff, relationship to board, and board support function.

The brochure sets the stage for more comprehensive training of board members in the future. The chief executive officer or board members conducting the recruitment interview can use the brochure as a discussion document during the interview.

This practice will enable the center to recruit board members who understand their role and who come prepared to receive further training.

BOARD ORIENTATION

A board orientation program should be provided for all new board members. New board members are eager to learn more about their assumed responsibilities and are receptive and amenable to adapting themselves to the defined role.

CONTENT OF ORIENTATION PROGRAM

A common mistake of orientation programs is that the entire orientation is committed to explaining the agency's programs and services. Little time is committed to explaining the new board member's role.

An orientation program should acquaint new board members with the center, the community mental health center movement, the work of community mental health centers, and the responsibilities of governing boards. A basic program outline should include:

1. *History of Community Mental Health*: Explain the beginnings and purpose of community mental health. Although there have been significant changes in the mental health industry, it is important for new board members to understand the historical and philosophical background that led to where centers are today.
2. *History of the Local Center*: Provide a history of the center, its services, funding, role in the community, and organizational structure. This topic should be sufficient to enable board members to understand the center, but it should not be the dominant topic of the orientation.
3. *The Purpose of Citizen Boards*: Explain the historical rationale for the use of citizen/lay boards in community mental health centers. Clarify that citizens are not selected as board members for their expertise in mental health, management, finance, marketing, or personnel, but for their knowledge of the community.
4. *The Responsibilities of Governing Boards*: Explain the role of the governing board, what it is supposed to do, and how the board is organized. An abbreviated form of Board Training Program No. 1 (presented later in this chapter) may be used for the orientation.
5. *Working with the Executive Director*: Explain the role of the executive, how it differs from the board role, and how executive and board work together. This is an especially important time to clarify the roles so that role confusion can be prevented.

WHO SHOULD CONDUCT
THE ORIENTATION PROGRAM?

The chief executive officer should conduct this orientation program and thereby demonstrate his or her leadership. Other staff members or board members may be included in the program, but the chief executive must clearly be in command and control of the program. If it seems important for the board chairperson to have a more prominent role, the chief executive officer and board chair could jointly conduct the orientation.

The only circumstances that would warrant an outside trainer for the orientation program is where the chief executive officer's credibility is seriously in question.

TIME FOR THE ORIENTATION PROGRAM

Conduct the orientation before new members are actually seated on the board. If this is not possible, conduct the orientation as soon as possible after they are seated.

The orientation program must be conducted at a time when all new board members can attend. Allocate a full day to allow time to cover all subjects thoroughly. If board members work during the week, a weekend may be the best option.

All board members should be encouraged to attend the orientation. This enables the executive to introduce them to the new board members and provides a refresher training course for old board members.

FORMAL BOARD TRAINING

Informal board training has its place, but nothing takes the place of formal board training. Assure that the board receives at least one formal board training program each year. The program content can vary from year to year to maintain interest, but the training should not be neglected. The training is so important that some boards require members to receive training on a continuous basis in order to retain board membership.

SECURING BOARD SUPPORT FOR TRAINING

Board members sometimes resist board training. The resistance often stems from the implied suggestion that they are incompetent to perform their board roles. Some board members will cite the number of boards on which they have served or their years of experience as a board member as evidence of their knowledge of board governance.

Resistance must be overcome before an effective board training program can be established. Board members must recognize the need, want the training, and participate fully in order for the program to be successful.

An approach that has been used effectively in some centers to reduce the resistance is to take the focus off the board. A presentation can be made to the board identifying the need for continuing education and training for both board and staff. A strong case can be made for upgrading skills of everyone involved at the governance level, management level, clinical level, and support level. If the presentation is made by the executive, he or she can emphasize his or her own need for ongoing training. The desired goal is a board policy on training at all levels.

BUDGETING BOARD TRAINING

If ongoing board training is an agenda for the center, a financial commitment must be made as a budget item. Training methods will have some costs, and the costs should be planned and budgeted. The allocated amount should include the direct training costs and any out-of-pocket expenses to be incurred by board members such as travel, food, and lodging.

Boards may allocate money for staff training but often are unwilling to commit money to train themselves. Board members often believe that spending money for their own training is self-serving. Considering the board must be convinced that board training is probably one of the best investments the center could make, the board must recognize the center's obligation to pay for governing board training.

WHAT TYPE OF BOARD TRAINING?

Generic training for not-for-profit boards is available in many cities and through a number of national organizations. The training has value but is not directed to the specific issues of community mental health centers.

Formal board training programs are available at many state and national mental health conferences. The National Council of Community Mental Health Centers conducts a Board Leadership Conference each year at its annual meeting. Some state associations provide formal board training at their meetings. The programs offer an assortment of training opportunities that focus on community mental health center boards. However, unless these programs are held locally, attendance by board members is difficult.

An ideal option is to provide training that is specifically tailored to the needs, problems, and issues of a single governing board. Many community mental health centers have been successful in reshaping the entire operation of their governance function through such training programs. The key to success is to include all board members in the training, address issues that are directly applicable to the board's training needs, create a plan to incorporate the new information into board practices, and establish a method to monitor progress.

179

WHEN TO CONDUCT FORMAL BOARD TRAINING

Board members usually have limited time and expect that their time be used efficiently. They appreciate training that can be combined with regular board meetings. Informal training can and should be included in all board meetings, as indicated earlier in this chapter. However, attempting to compress a formal training agenda into a regular board meeting is likely to reduce the effectiveness of both the training and the business meeting.

The most successful programs have occurred when a block of time has been set aside solely for board training. Designate a slot each year on the board calendar for a training seminar or workshop. Board members will learn to expect it and participate.

Undertaking a board training program of substance requires at least a 6-hour block of time. Some centers have found that one and one-half days provides the greatest benefit. In any case, there should be enough time to cover the topics comfortably without the feeling of being rushed.

WHERE TO CONDUCT FORMAL BOARD TRAINING

Some centers conduct board training in the board room where the board normally conducts its meetings. If the training budget is low, this may be the best option, particularly if the room is conducive to training.

Other centers select settings away from the center, such as professional training sites, hotels, conference centers, universities, or churches. If the training program is to last longer than 1 day, a lodge, resort, retreat center, or hotel may be a logical choice. A weekend training program can allow time for socialization as well as training.

WHO SHOULD CONDUCT THE BOARD TRAINING?

This question usually must be prefaced by three other questions: What is the budget for training? Is there someone in-house who is a competent board trainer? If there is someone in-house, does that person have the credibility with the board to assume a teaching role?

If the training budget allows, bring in an outsider who is an experienced professional in board training. This practice generally assures a quality training program and allows the executive and board members to relax and participate in the training.

If the budget does not permit outside help, however, inside resources may be used. An executive experienced in board training may conduct the training. This arrangement may be particularly suitable if the executive is relatively new to the job. It gives the executive an opportunity to express ideas to the board and begin building a good working relationship. If the executive has been in the position for considerable time or has conducted training for the board several times previously, though, it may be more advantageous to use someone else for the training.

The center may have an experienced board member who is adept at conducting board training programs. If respected by the board, this person may be the logical choice.

The remainder of this chapter provides outlines of two board-training programs. These outlines provide a basic framework and may be used by an in-house presenter in developing the instructional material.

BOARD TRAINING PROGRAM NO. 1

This is a basic board training program for new or inexperienced board members but may be repeated periodically for older board members. It is designed to provide board members with practical information on general issues of required board activity. This training session should focus on the routine business of what the board actually is supposed to do and how it is to be done. The program can be structured to increase the skills of board members. The program takes about 4 to 6 hours for presentation.

PLANNING: DECIDING WHAT IS TO BE DONE

A primary responsibility of the board is planning or deciding the organization's goals and objectives. This is an ongoing task and should occupy a major portion of the board's time.

Planning is not a popular concept in many organizations because of the bureaucratic manner in which it has been approached in the past. Often much time has been spent developing elaborate goals, objectives, and strategies that were designed to meet the requirements of a funding source and may be unrelated to what actually goes on in the organization. These plans make attractive books to fill the shelves, but they have little value for the organization. Each organization needs instead a clear plan to give direction and guide decision making. Without a plan the organization flounders and is without focus.

Planning must occur at all levels of the organization and is a shared responsibility of board and staff. This section clarifies the planning role of the board; it can be used to help the board members begin to develop a long-range approach to planning. The board's real value is in shaping the future of the organization rather than focusing on the present.

Planning at the board level consists of the following activities:

1. *Defining the Philosophy:* The board is responsible for defining and periodically reviewing the organizational philosophy. The community mental health center exists as an organization because of certain beliefs and values about community needs and the services that should be provided to meet those needs. The organizational philosophy is a statement of the underlying beliefs and values upon which the organization is based and will influence all decisions of the center.

   If the philosophy is not clearly articulated, board members and staff members may operate on different assumptions about what the organization should be doing. This leads to various components of the center working in conflict with each other.

2. *Establishing the Mission or Purpose:* The board is responsible for establishing and periodically reviewing the organizational mission. The mission or purpose statement defines the nature of the business. The statement grows out of the philosophy and condenses into a single statement the reason for the existence of the organization. It becomes the basic frame of reference for all decisions about what the organization will do.

3. *Reviewing Community Needs and Preferences:* The board is responsible for reviewing the existing community needs or problems that fall within the scope of the agency's mission.

   The board is not responsible for conducting needs assessments or market research (this is staff work), but the board must review the results of these efforts in order to establish organizational goals.

4. *Setting Goals:* The board is responsible for determining the major organizational goals that the center will attempt to attain. The goals should be long range, in order

to give the board more control of the destiny of the organization and steer activities toward the future. Short-term goals affect the day-to-day management and are best left for management to decide.

The board's goals should be stated in terms of outcome rather than process. The board must decide what the organization is expected to accomplish.

5. *Review and Approval of Plan:* Although the board is responsible for the final review and approval of the organizational plan, the plan is actually developed by staff under the direction of the chief executive officer. Based on the philosophy, mission statement, and goals established by the board, staff will develop objectives, strategies, time frames, and measurements. The final plan will be presented to the board.

POLICY DEVELOPMENT: DECIDING HOW IT WILL BE DONE

Policy development is a primary responsibility of the board. After the board has established its goals and approved its plan, the board must develop policies to communicate how decisions are to be made in the implementation of the plan. Since the board obviously cannot make all decisions within the organization, it must provide guidance to those who will make the day-to-day decisions.

A policy is a broad statement designed to guide decision making to assure that the organization's goals are achieved and that decisions are made consistently. It is a tool used by the board to govern the organization.

The process of policy development includes the following steps:

1. *Policy Issue Identification:* From time to time issues are identified within the center that require management decisions. If there is no policy to authorize or guide a decision, it must be taken to the board. Since the underlying issue is likely to arise again in the future, it is wise to establish a policy on the issue so that it will not require board action each time. When the issue is identified, it is taken to the appropriate board committee.
2. *Policy Planning:* When the issue is presented to the board committee, the committee must plan whether a

policy is needed, and if so, what the policy will be. The policy planning process includes an evaluation of options. The role of staff during this process is to provide any needed information.

3. *Policy Formulation:* When the committee has agreed on the basic content of the policy, someone must write the policy. It is wise to have one person develop the wording of the policy based on the committee's agreement. The writing of the policy is usually a staff responsibility.

4. *Policy Approval:* After the policy is written, it must be presented to the full board by the committee for approval.

5. *Policy Issuance:* After the policy is approved by the board, it must be issued to all parties that are affected.

The policy then becomes an official document to be used by management in decision making. Detailed procedures for implementation of the policy may be developed and issued by staff with the approval of the chief executive officer.

DELEGATION: DECIDING WHO WILL DO IT

Delegation is the process used by the board for formally granting authority and responsibility to others for implementing its plan in accordance with its policies. It is a process of empowerment.

Although the board may choose to delegate to others, most delegation is to three categories:

1. *Chief Executive Officer:* The board must have a formal process for official delegation of authority and responsibility for the management of the center to its executive. Without this delegation, the board retains all authority, and the organization cannot operate.

   Clarify the distinction between the board/governance role and the executive/management role at this point in the training.

2. *Board Officers and Committees:* The board must decide what authority and responsibility it chooses to grant to its officers and committees.

3. *Contractors:* In some situations the board may choose to delegate certain authority and responsibilities to outside contractors such as attorneys and accountants.

The training program should include a thorough discussion of how and to whom delegation will occur.

FINANCING: DECIDING
WHO WILL PAY FOR IT

The board is responsible for the financing of the operations of the center. The board must decide where and how the funds will be obtained. Boards sometimes neglect this responsibility and leave it to staff. Staff can certainly implement the board's decisions, but the board must take responsibility for determining how it chooses to finance the center's operation.

The board is also responsible for determining how the funds will be allocated (budget) and spent (financial policies) in carrying out its plan.

MONITORING: MEASURING
WHAT HAS BEEN DONE

Once the board has developed its plan, determined its policies, delegated responsibility, and established financing, it has a responsibility to monitor whether these things are being done. The most common method used is staff and committee reports provided to the board. If the board is to monitor effectively, it must receive reports with the right information.

A common error in many community mental health centers is to provide the board with reports that were prepared for funders or governmental bodies. The reports are often confusing and distracting for board members because they do not contain the information needed by the board and have much extraneous information. As a result, the board members ask the wrong questions.

Most financial reports provide a reporting of line item expenditures. These reports offer little meaningful information for boards to evaluate, but it often leads them to ask questions about line item expenditures. Reporting income and expenditures by program category works better.

Board members seldom know the kind of information to request. Often there is too much information to be useful. It may be advantageous for the executive to spend time trying to determine the type of information that would be most useful for the board in determining whether its goals are being attained and its policies implemented.

EVALUATION: ASSESSING THE
VALUE OF WHAT HAS BEEN DONE

Board members are often confused by the idea of evaluation. The confusion probably stems from the fact that evaluation reports are usually presented to them in very technical terms that are not understandable. This highly technical approach to evaluation may be appropriate for the professional evaluator, but it seldom works with boards.

The board's role in evaluation can be as simple as comparing what has been done with what the board directed to be done. If the board has received the appropriate reports, it should not be difficult to determine whether the goals have been attained, the policies were implemented, expenditures were in line with allocations, the executive carried out the direction of the board, and the board performed the tasks that it assigned to itself.

If the board feels the need for further evaluation of specific areas, a consultant or professional evaluator may be hired to perform the task.

BOARD TRAINING PROGRAM NO. 2

This program could be entitled *Building Sound Board Relationships.* The program is for seasoned boards trying to improve overall effectiveness. The training identifies important constituent groups, defines the potential nature of the relationships, and describes possible problems and opportunities in those relationships. The program assists boards in understanding how to build and sustain productive relationships with various constituent groups.

A community mental health center board makes decisions that have impact on and are judged by many constituent groups. Each group will from time to time have serious concerns about decisions made by the board. As the number, size, and diversity of these constituent groups increase, so too will the potential for conflicting demands.

The board must clearly define its relationship with each constituent group. The board must listen to the issues and concerns of each group and determine how the information is incorporated into the board's decision-making process. Equally important, the board must determine how to provide information to each constituent group.

An outline for instructors follows. The outline may be customized to a local board's needs.

BOARD - EXECUTIVE DIRECTOR RELATIONSHIP

The board's relationship with its executive director is probably its most important relationship. If this relationship is based on clear role definition, mutual trust, and competent role performance, the board and executive can work together to resolve most other issues. An impaired relationship is likely to have a negative impact in every level of the organization.

This segment of the program helps the board members understand the benefits of a positive working relationship with the executive. If problems currently exist in the relationship, the program provides an opportunity to explore the problems and define a solution.

There are three primary ingredients to a positive working relationship between board and executive director. Problems usually occur when a breakdown occurs in any of these three areas:

1. *Role Clarification:* Most problems between boards and their executives stem from role confusion. Training Program No. 1 dealt to some extent with the clarification of roles. This program offers an opportunity to reinforce that clarification. A clear and understandable distinction must exist between management (executive director) and governance (board). The distinction must carry the authority of formal board policy in order to be effective. The references at the end of this chapter include several articles that speak to this distinction.

2. *Mutual Trust:* Trust between a board and its executive is generally based on clear and open communication between the board and the executive. Problems often arise when information is withheld (or an impression is left that information is being withheld) by board or executive.

   Boards rely upon the executive for information about issues that board members consider significant. The mere hint that information is being withheld erodes trust. Boards do not like to be surprised by a crisis. This training program explores the type of information the board needs from its executive to make governance decisions.

Boards sometimes appear to withhold information from the executive. This usually occurs when the board, committees, or board members hold meetings that exclude the executive. Even when such meetings have a positive intent, they tend to erode trust. There are few issues that the board and executive cannot discuss openly and frankly.

3. *Performance:* The board has a right to expect satisfactory performance by the executive. Yet, the board must specify its expectations of the executive and periodically evaluate performance based on those expectations. This part of the program provides an opportunity for the board to discuss expectations and to decide upon a process for cvaluation.

Equally important, if the board fails to provide policy guidance and support to its executive, the relationship may break down. The board must also establish performance expectations for itself and periodically rate its own performance.

The instructor should use this section of the training program to encourage the board and executive to identify specific areas where the relationship can be improved.

BOARD - STAFF RELATIONSHIP

The board is responsible to assure that the relationship between the board and staff is based on mutual respect and support. The appropriate board-staff relationship is a formal one with formal channels that build and maintain the relationship. The executive director is the vital connection linking the board and staff. If either board members or staff members circumvent that channel, they undermine the organizational structure and damage the system.

It is not suggested that direct relationships between board members and staff members should be completely avoided. In smaller communities board and staff members are often neighbors or friends. In larger organizations, staff members are often assigned responsibility for staffing board committees. However, it must be emphasized that these informal relationships do not substitute for the official relationship between the board and staff. Informal relationships should not muddle the role of the executive as the link between board and staff.

Board members must recognize that their position may intimidate staff members. As a result, staff members may feel compelled to respond directly to every suggestion or question by a board member as if it were a requirement. Conversely, some clever staff members may use board members to undermine the role of the executive and cause dissension between the board and executive.

This section of the training session can be used to aid the board in developing a policy or position statement that defines the relationship between board and staff.

BOARD - FUNDER RELATIONSHIP

The relationship between the center and its major funder is one of the most important of all relationships with which the board must be concerned. Funders, whether state, county, local, or regional governmental authority, have formidable influence on the survival of the center. One of the board's most significant duties is to focus on the funder-center relationship.

Some community mental health centers are operated directly by governmental bodies, and their boards are simply advisory in nature. More frequently, however, centers are private, not-for-profit organizations that relate to the funding body by contractual agreement. In a contractual relationship, the funder provides funding and imposes certain requirements, and the center provides services to the community.

Although some funding bodies encourage centers to become stronger and more independent by seeking additional sources of funding, other funders have not been able to grow beyond the parental role. They attempt to foster dependency by controlling all center resources and activities. The relationship between a community mental health center and its funding body often evolves as a parent-child relationship.

When faced with controlling funders, mental health center boards often feel intimidated and powerless to make decisions about the center and its future. Boards within such centers often accept the dependent child role and reluctantly abdicate the role of responsibility for decision making for the mental health center. Often, such boards fail to establish financial reserves for their centers and become even more dependent on the funder for all decisions.

Other center boards may develop adversarial relationships with funders. These boards often make demands of funders without recognizing the concerns and needs of the funding agency, leading to a pattern of rebellion and continual conflict with funders.

A responsible mental health center board recognizes that it is, in fact, directly responsible for the center and its future, regardless of the current relationship or degree of dependency on its funder. A responsible board will respect the role of its funder but will also develop a long-range strategy for the financial strength and viability of the center.

A mental heath center board should relate to its funder as a commercial business relates to an important customer. The funder is buying a service from the center and the center must assure that the funder is satisfied with the service. Whether a state, county, city, or other, the funder usually wants to pay for a particular service to a particular population. To assure continuation of funds, the board must determine the goals, needs and preferences of funders and assure that the service is provided to the funder's satisfaction.

The board must remember that the funding agency must also account for its use of public money. The funder cannot simply give money to a center without some form of accountability.

A primary concern of most funding agencies is determining whether the money allocated is spent for the purpose intended. To make this determination, funders place restrictions on centers and require accounts, reports, audits, and site visits. Yet, usually, the funder does not know what is happening in the center. The information passed to the funder does not adequately convey information about the value of programs and the quality of services.

The board can strengthen its relationship with the funding agency by providing clear and useful information to the funder. When funding decisions are made, funders are likely to give more money to centers they best understand.

BOARD - CONSUMER RELATIONSHIP

A community mental health center exists primarily to provide services to consumers who need services. Primary consumers, secondary consumers, and potential consumers constitute a dominant constituent group that is often concerned about the decisions and actions of the center's governing board. The board must clearly understand its appropriate role in relating to consumers.

190

Zealous board members sometimes have a tendency to become overly concerned about individual consumers, their treatment approach, and their personal reaction to the center's services. This situation occurs often when board members are deeply committed to serving people but are unclear about the role of the agency board. Board members who make misguided attempts to help individual consumers frequently risk breaches of confidentiality, disruption of the service delivery system, and disservice to the consumer.

Another common error of boards is the tendency to distance themselves from consumer issues by refusing to address consumer concerns. When approached by consumer groups, boards may even become defensive or protective of the agency rather than being open-minded and objective.

The board should cultivate and maintain formal relationships with groups or associations of consumers and family members. These relationships should focus on broad issues of general concern to consumers and families rather than individual treatment issues. Input from consumer groups can be valuable to boards in developing agency policy.

This part of the training program can provide both positive and negative examples of board involvement with consumer issues.

BOARD - COMMUNITY RELATIONSHIP

A community mental health center is a community agency and has a fundamental responsibility to serve the best interests of the general community as well as primary consumers. In some cases the center may be dependent upon the goodwill of the community for much of its financial support. The center's public image and community support are vital to success.

Board members (community residents) are the link between the center and the community. Most board members recognize this fact and are sensitive to community comments and attitudes about the center. Board members often represent the center to the community and provide community input to policy decision making. In times of crisis, board members may even serve as a buffer between the center and the community.

Boards must give priority to the relationship between the center and the community. Boards must take a proactive posture in building a strong positive image in the community for the center, but they also must be prepared to react creatively to negative

191

issues that arise. Communities are composed of various factions or special interest groups with conflicting needs, desires, and demands. Occasionally, there are conflicts between the needs and desires of community groups and the best interests of consumers of the center's services. The responsible board will be alert to the conflicting demands of differing constituent groups and will make clear its role and relationship with the community.

This training offers an opportunity for the board to define its desired relationship with the community and how this relationship is developed and maintained. The inevitable crises in community relations can be weathered if the board has created in advance the public image it intends to project, the relationship it hopes to maintain with the community, and how issues of public confidence and public demand will be handled.

BOARD - MEDIA RELATIONSHIP

The center's relationship with the mass media is a part of its relationship with the community but requires special treatment in this training program. The media are a powerful force and can have great influence (either positive or negative) upon the center's relationship with the community. The board must always be conversant in its relationship with the media.

Some centers exist for a considerable time with little or no exposure to the media except an occasional news item about a particular program or event. Yet an unanticipated adverse incident or controversy may thrust the center into the forefront of news coverage without time for planning. In many situations board members may find themselves unprepared and vulnerable to negative publicity.

The issue of board-media relations is too important to be left to chance. The board should plan its desired media relations in advance of direct contact with the media. The board should designate an individual who is authorized to speak to the media for the center and for the board. This practice avoids the potential of conflicting statements by different board members.

PROGRAM FOLLOW-UP

The conclusion of the training program can include a discussion of how the board will define its working relationships with each of its constituent groups. Perhaps an assignment can be made to each of the board committees to work on developing a proposed policy statement on the board's relationship with one of its constituent groups.

Following the discussion, a follow-up should be planned that formally defines the board's major relationships. Without formal follow-up, the potential impact of the training may be partially lost.

CONCLUSION

Proficient boards are seldom created by coincidence. Expertise in governance usually is the result of recurrent training and seasoned experience. A periodic assessment of board training needs and a systematic training plan can strengthen the entire organization.

The training of board members must be a high priority for the executive director. Only the chief executive is in a position to guide the process of building an informed, well-trained board. If this prime responsibility is neglected, the executive may spend his or her time trying to repair the damage caused by the neglect.

The opportunities to provide training for board members are unlimited. A skillful executive director will be alert to each opportunity, will provide or facilitate appropriate training, and will continue to augment board effectiveness.

James O. Gibson, MSW, is currently Chairman of GibsonFisher Ltd., a national healthcare consulting firm based in Columbus, Ohio. The company specializes in providing management and governance consulting for mental health programs. Mr. Gibson has had extensive experience in working with mental health centers and their governing boards. Mr. Gibson may be contacted at GibsonFisher Ltd., 550 East Town Street, Columbus, OH 43215.

REFERENCES

The following references may be of value to the training leader in preparation of programs:

Berger, S., & Sudman, S. K. (1989, May-June). Successful CEOs read warning signs. *Healthcare Executive, 4,* 22-24.

Burdett, R. J., Jr. (1989, May-June). The five commandments of governance. *Healthcare Executive, 4,* 27-28.

Carver, J. (1980, October). *Board Leadership on Nonprofit Boards* (Board Practices Monograph No. 12). Washington, DC: National Association of Corporate Directors.

CEO-Board Relations. (1989, April 5). *Hospitals,* pp. 38-42.

Chait, R. P., & Taylor, B. E. (1989, January-February). Charting the territory of nonprofit boards. *Harvard Business Review,* pp. 44-54.

Cleverley, W. O. (1989, May-June). How boards can use comparative data in strategic planning. *Healthcare Executive, 4,* 32-33.

Gill, S. L. (1989, May-June). Patterns and trends in healthcare governance. *Healthcare Executive, 4,* 20-21.

Hart, J. D., & Hageman, W. M. (1989, May-June). Streamlining your corporate structure: A new concept in governance. *Healthcare Executive, 4,* 25-26.

Institute for Voluntary Organizations. (1978). *Self-Diagnosis Guidelines for Voluntary Governing Boards of Directors.* Chicago, IL: Author.

National Institute of Mental Health. (1979). *Orientation Manual for Citizen Boards of Federally Funded Community Mental Health Centers* (DHEW Publication No. ADM 78-759). Washington DC: U.S. Government Printing Office.

Peterfreund, N. (1980, Fall). *Community Mental Health Center Manual for Board Development.* Washington, DC: U.S. Government Printing Office.

Price, W. (1977). *Manual on Governance and Policy Planning for CMHC Board Members.* Silver Springs, MD: Wolfgang Price Associates.

Smith, B. V. (1987, Fall). Community mental health center governance: A study of board chairpersons and CEOs. *Journal of Mental Health Administration, 14,* 14-19.

Uterman, I., & Davis, R. H. (1982, May-June). The strategy gap in not-for profits. *Harvard Business Review,* pp. 30-34.

Management Styles:
Making a
Good Match Fit

Timothy H. Lentner
and Saul Cooper

Is it truly possible for one to "choose" a management style? Or are we already "chosen" by our personalities, life experiences, and the environment of the organization in which we work? Clinicians debate whether one can "change" by making conscious choices or only through long-term, in-depth psychotherapy, or by some other means that focuses intensely on our styles of thinking and behaving.

The problem for today's administrators and managers is that most find themselves in a new position because it presented an opportunity for advancement, and few other choices were - or were perceived to be - available to them. There is a wealth of literature (see your daily junk mail and myriad workshops) in the administrative/management arena, each expert hawking his or her wares as the ultimate solution to everyone's management problems. Management "style" must be the problem, and he or she has the solution.

The assumption seems to be made that the "ideal" management style exists out there somewhere and that one's life or career goal should be to find and adopt that style. This might be referred to as the "golden fleece" style of management or living. However, there are other images that may more accurately describe the process of a manager's search for a style that "fits" with the organization, its goals, and oneself as an individual.

The perception of the existence of an "ideal" management style may be linked to another general perception in both professional and lay circles. That is the perception of an ideal personality style toward which one ought to strive. This value has been reinforced through centuries of archetypal religious teaching and decades of psychological training as well as other forms of socialization within our society.

However, there is a strong case to be made for a different understanding of that process, both in one's personal life and in one's professional career - the difference between the two being almost imperceptible at times. Jung provides an image of "wholeness" through the concept of the "self" that administrators or managers may find well worth exploring (Jung, 1959).

As individuals, we are made up of many conflicting feelings, styles, values, and directions within our lives. We have many different interests with varying strengths and weaknesses, all of which are not necessarily consonant with each other. The search for wholeness cannot eliminate all conflict and disagreement. These "opposites" within are understood as strengths that can be integrated into an individual (Jung, 1959). The ideal integration brings about "wholeness," an integrated "self."

The most important part, for our purposes, is that this search for wholeness is different for each individual. And although there are some general principles that might be considered "ideal" for all to strive toward, one's ability to figure out which differences will "fit" and which will not is critical for the success of a person in a particular management position.

We will set forth generally accepted management principles that bring about predictable consequences. However, we would pose this question: Is it possible to evaluate in advance the variables of a potential management position and make a reasonably accurate projection of whether one's present management style would "fit" with the new organization or department, or would bring about more discord than either individual or organization would find acceptable?

Any individual considering a new management position already has a history of managing people and situations (job, home, social environment) developed over many years, even decades. A similar history exists on the side of the organization. The agency within which that position exists most likely has a history that spans many years in one form or another. Patterns have developed on both sides that have become ingrained in each and have become the basis upon which any action is evaluated. A "change" in management style, either through hiring a person with a new perspective that departs from all previous histories or through efforts to adopt a new management style described by pertinent literature, may or may not work effectively depending on how it affects "the fit" between those histories.

In sum, we believe that success depends on an effective fit between the basic assumption of the organization and the style of the manager.

PRINCIPLES FOR
EFFECTIVE STAFF MANAGEMENT

Here we will review some general management principles that serve as a foundation for our thinking. Then, we will suggest some principles and a checklist that can serve as a guide for evaluating "the fit" with a new position.

For the past two decades we have heard multiple points of view on the subject of "What really motivates staff?" "Recognition" and "praise" have been dominant themes, which also happen to fit with our mental health value systems. Typically, "money" has been a distant second. However, two recent studies suggest that these values are beginning to change (Adia Personnel Services, 1989; Locke, 1988). In both studies, employees surveyed ranked "money" as the primary motivator.

However, before confirming such a shift, we would do well to remember that multiple factors influence the performance of any given individual on any given job. The value of staff involvement and participation in problem solving, decision making, and goal setting has long been accepted in the mental health field as a primary motivator. It is through involvement in a genuine sharing of decision-making authority that people become invested in their work and motivated to deliver the best service possible. Opportunity for creative participation in the direction and work of the organization is in direct proportion to a person's investment in the work of the agency.

Therefore, it appears to us that a combination of a genuine recognition of staff competence, a meaningful sharing of decision-making authority, and a judicious use of "bonuses" directly related to the productive use of the sharing of that authority are the most effective motivators. These factors are quite different from the appearance of power, image building, surge for status, and money that is commonly "hyped" through the articles of many of the popular management magazines and training brochures.

This, however, does not mean that all administrators and organizations accept the values that we are espousing and operate in that manner. The issue of one's authority and how to use it is perhaps the single most frequent dynamic with which an administrator or manager struggles. The use and misuse of that authority is critical to finding that elusive management style commonly hyped today.

The whole issue of whether and how one decides to share that authority with staff is firmly rooted in one's degree of comfort with authority, a willingness to take risks, a tolerance for ambiguity, and an ability to evaluate and trust those with whom one shares that decision-making authority. This implies that the manager must come to grips honestly with a broad range of authority issues.

A further point of contention is the basic question of whether one can share or delegate the "responsibility" as well as the "authority." We take the firm position that an administrator or manager must be held responsible for all aspects of the decisions made by those to whom he or she has delegated that authority. One cannot give away the responsibility along with the authority and remain a responsible manager. This is all part of the risk involved when deciding whether to share that decision and planning authority with others.

There always will be those who perceive the delegation of authority as a means of "passing the buck," "ducking," or taking "the easy way out" of fulfilling one's assigned responsibilities. We believe that this perception generally comes from those who are not comfortable with the degree of risk taking required and who therefore tend to exercise their authority in a safer and more autocratic manner. We further suggest that these are the actions of an administrator or manager who has not yet learned the wealth of good ideas that can come from the collective efforts of others. They often perceive this type of action as a potentially negative reflection upon their own competence. Comfort with authority is in direct proportion to comfort with oneself.

Administrators or managers must, therefore, take into account an accurate assessment of their own management history before considering any job. Questions they must ask themselves are: What is my level of tolerance for ambiguity? What is my ability to take risks? How comfortable am I with the responsibility of having authority over others? How comfortable am I with the responsibility of evaluating and trusting someone else's skill and expertise in doing something for which I will ultimately be held responsible?

Similar questions need to be asked regarding the expectations of the use of that authority on the part of the agency or organization in which I will be functioning in my next job. What are the values, expectations, and history of those to whom I will be held responsible? What is the style by which they set the tone of the agency? What are the values, expectations, and history of those I will supervise, those who will be looking to me for leadership and authority?

A MANAGEMENT STYLE CHECKLIST

The checklist on pages 204-207 is intended to offer an informal means of assessing one's own management style and expectations in relation to those of the organization or department in which the new job is located. It is not a formal instrument; there are no data concerning its reliability or validity. It can, however, serve as an informal basis for considering "the fit" between you and a new job, differences that are worthy of note. It may suggest areas that need negotiation. And it may serve as an indicator of potential problem areas as you proceed through the decision-making process when approaching a job change.

HOW TO USE THE CHECKLIST

The Administrator/Manager/Supervisor section of the "Self Assessment" scale, and the Organization/Department segment of the "Job Assessment" scale are each a series of 25 questions intended to solicit information in five areas which are pivotal to understanding organizational dynamics. These five areas are as follows:

1. *Decision-Making Style*: Understanding of, and comfort with, one's own authority has a direct impact on how decisions are made. Each assessment form has five questions designed to evoke an evaluation of both individual and organizational dynamics from authoritarian to an egalitarian model.
2. *Risk-Taking Behaviors*: Decision-making, program planning, staff supervision, and a host of other management and organizational functions are characterized by certain behaviors which can be described according to "risk." For example, risk taking may involve the individual (or organization) engaging in a mode of operating (decisions, choices, sharing authority, etc.) which depends on someone else's ability to achieve the desired goal for

which you are held responsible. Or, it might be a behavior in which an "unorthodox" set of procedures are designed to accomplish the desired result. Each assessment form has five questions designed to evaluate the tendency to engage in risk-taking behaviors.

3. *Ambiguity Factors*: A person's ability to tolerate ambiguity in a complex organization is in direct relationship to his or her decision-making style and risk-taking behavior. The organization or department, as a reflection of its history and staff attributes, operates with its own level of toleration for ambiguity. Each assessment has five questions designed to solicit that degree of tolerance.

4. *Delegating Style*: Delegating is a more specific factor within one's style of decision making. It is a primary variable in describing how decisions are made within an organization. Each assessment has five questions designed to elicit information about how the individual or organization feels about delegating authority and responsibility.

5. *Lifestyle Factors*: Just as there are individuals who never consider how the quality of their lives will be affected by a new job, there are also organizations who could not care less. However, lifestyle issues have serious implications for any individual considering a change in position. It is one of the major factors leading to unhappiness, stress, and eventual "burnout." Likewise, organizations are becoming more sensitive to these issues if they want to keep their employees longer, keep efficiency levels high, and encourage innovative thinking. Each assessment has five questions designed to draw out factors that may be significant.

Note: Questions on one assessment are matched to the other assessment by checking the question number and the abbreviation code on Table 1 (p. 201) and Table 2 (p. 202). For example, question number 2 on the Self Assessment scale is coded "5-Amb" which matches question number 5 on the Job Assessment scale, coded "2-Amb."

DIRECTIONS FOR
COMPLETING CHECKLISTS

Place a check mark under "Agree" or "Disagree" on each question of the Self Assessment and Job Assessment scales (see

TABLE 1: QUESTION CATEGORIES

NUMBER OF QUESTIONS IN EACH CATEGORY	ABBREVIATIONS	CATEGORIES
5	D	Decision-Making Style
5	R	Risk-Taking Behaviors
5	Amb	Ambiguity Factors
5	Del	Delegating Style
5	L	Lifestyle Factors

pages 204-207). The questions require forced choices that do not allow for variations in order to list a clear profile by category, so use the choice that most clearly reflects your answer.

The Job Assessment scale addresses information to be collected by an individual considering a new position. The Self Assessment scale provides the same opportunity when used by the interviewing organization/department. Gathering complete information in order to accurately fill out the "other" assessment may be difficult. However, when organizations and potential managers assess each other, they are involved in making these kinds of determinations. These checklists can be used to enhance the information collected during the interview process.

SCORING DIRECTIONS

After completing both assessment instruments, fill in the "Score By Question Form" (p. 208) indicating the number of questions matched by category. For example, compare the answer to question number 2 on the Self Assessment scale to question number 5 (corresponding question, see Table 2) on the Job Assessment scale. If they match, put a check mark in the "Match" column on the "Score By Question Form."

Next, transfer the score to the "Total Matches By Category Form" (p. 209). The "Question Number" columns are the numbers of the questions on the Self Assessment scale. If you had a "match" scored on the "Score By Question Form," put a check

---

TABLE 2: CATEGORY KEY

CATEGORY	QUESTION NUMBER	
	Self Assessment	*Job Assessment*
Decision-Making Style	1	1
	5	20
	10	3
	12	23
	15	19
Risk Taking Behaviors	6	9
	8	21
	16	14
	17	13
	23	24
Ambiguity Factors	2	5
	4	8
	11	12
	18	2
	20	16
Delegating Style	3	6
	9	17
	14	11
	21	22
	24	25
Lifestyle Factors	7	4
	13	10
	19	15
	22	7
	25	18

---

mark in the corresponding field on the "Total Matches By Category Form." Leave blank any that do not match. Total the number of check marks by column (categories) and figure the percentage of match. Add the category totals to arrive at Total Score and Total Percentage.

INTERPRETING THE RESULTS

The resulting scores will provide a straightforward means of reviewing questions to be considered as one decides upon a potential career move. Readers should evaluate the match or mismatch of a given category according to their perception of its relative importance for them. Obviously, all of us are different and may weigh the trade-offs differently depending on our life and career goals.

We caution that we are providing an organized means of thinking about a new job and potential career advancement, not a scale by which one can predict success or failure in a new job. We offer no data to support the reliability or validity of these checklists.

From the agency's perspective, this profile tool may provide similar information in the review of candidates for managerial positions.

CONCLUSIONS

The "choice" of a management style and the accompanying movement into a particular job are often predetermined by an individual's personal and career histories and the history of the agency or department in which the job is located. The ability to assess the probability of how well one's style and values will fit with the needs of the agency may be a useful factor in making decisions for future job advancement and successful manager-organization matches.

MANAGEMENT STYLE CHECKLIST

ADMINISTRATOR/MANAGER/SUPERVISOR

SELF ASSESSMENT

AGREE	DISAGREE	
		(Check either "AGREE" or "DISAGREE" for each question.)
____	____	1. I tend to make the decisions and then "sell" the wisdom of my decisions to those who must implement them.
____	____	2. Policies and procedures are mostly useful in agencies that are hierarchal and therefore more predictable, unlike most mental health centers.
____	____	3. Whenever possible I delegate the work to be done.
____	____	4. I value highly the efficient functioning of the organization.
____	____	5. I have more confidence in my own expertise than in those under me.
____	____	6. I am able to assertively communicate my ideas to my superiors, even when their ideas are markedly different.
____	____	7. It is important that I have good friends at work.
____	____	8. I do not like uncertain situations, especially if I have to depend on others.
____	____	9. I feel that delegation, too often, is only a means of "passing the buck."
____	____	10. I feel that because I have been given the responsibility, I should assume the burden of that decision making.
____	____	11. A good work setting is one that is predictable and stable.
____	____	12. I am comfortable using a team model of decision making.
____	____	13. It is natural for me to combine my private and professional life.
____	____	14. I am a detail person.
____	____	15. I feel that decisions are of better quality if other people's ideas are a part of the process.

AGREE	DISAGREE	(Check either "AGREE" or "DISA-GREE" for each question.)
____	____	16. I value an agency that encourages creativity and flexibility in the performance of one's job.
____	____	17. I prefer being assertive with my ideas even if it brings about conflict with my colleagues.
____	____	18. I strongly prefer to have all the details of my job in a written job description with clear statements of authority and responsibility.
____	____	19. I don't mind putting in extra hours even though it occasionally interferes with my private life.
____	____	20. I prefer a work environment that allows me to set a flexible schedule and emphasizes the competent completion of my job responsibilities.
____	____	21. I worry about delegating work because it runs the risk of my losing control over process and product.
____	____	22. I do not attach much importance to the norms of wearing a particular mode of dress.
____	____	23. I prefer to do the job that is assigned and not seek out other potential responsibilities which may inhibit my ability to accomplish all tasks in a timely manner.
____	____	24. Delegation promotes personal and professional growth.
____	____	25. I need to work with supportive people in a positive emotional climate.

ORGANIZATION/DEPARTMENT

JOB ASSESSMENT

AGREE   DISAGREE   (Check either "AGREE" or "DISA-
GREE" for each question.)

_____   _____   1. This organization highly values people who are not afraid to make deci-
sions.

_____   _____   2. Job descriptions specify the clear extent of one's authority.

_____   _____   3. It is important that the organization's
leader is widely described as decisive
and persuasive.

_____   _____   4. The agency or department has a built-
in support system for staff and takes
the initiative to maintain such an environment.

_____   _____   5. Policies and procedures are written,
clear, and referred to in relevant decision-making matters.

_____   _____   6. Top managers appropriately delegate
work as a general administrative style.

_____   _____   7. Top managers are usually comfortable
with and supportive of those who do
not always agree with them.

_____   _____   8. Organizational efficiency is highly
valued.

_____   _____   9. Managers do not perceive strong disagreement from subordinates as a
lack of commitment to the agency.

_____   _____   10. The agency does not draw clear distinctions between professional and
private lives.

_____   _____   11. The organization emphasizes personal attention to detail as a critical
part of management jobs.

_____   _____   12. The organization or department has a
history of predictability and stability.

_____   _____   13. The organization encourages healthy
conflict.

_____   _____   14. Agency managers are respected for
their creativity and flexibility.

AGREE	DISAGREE	(Check either "AGREE" or "DISA-GREE" for each question.)
____	____	15. The agency expects its managers to put in extra hours whenever needed.
____	____	16. Schedules permit flex-time, focusing on the completion of the job as the most important goal.
____	____	17. Agency managers feel that the people to be trusted are the ones who do the work themselves.
____	____	18. The agency or department sets a positive tone that is evident in the friendly demeanor of the staff.
____	____	19. Management has a process designed for soliciting ideas from front-line and supervisory staff.
____	____	20. The organization or department has a history of assertively taking on new ventures, solving problems, and looking for creative programming.
____	____	21. It is important to the organization that assigned responsibilities are carried out in a specified manner which is usually dictated from above.
____	____	22. This organization expects an administrator or manager to automatically coordinate all decision making with other departments.
____	____	23. This agency values managers who are able to accept complex responsibilities, setting priorities as needed, in order to accomplish all tasks.
____	____	24. Delegation is practiced as a means of distributing the work load and utilizing others' competence.
____	____	25. Agency managers do not ask for input, although staff could offer suggestions without fear of sanction.

SCORE BY QUESTION FORM		
Questions Self / Job	Category (Abbrev)	Match (Check)
1 1	D	
2 5	Amb	
3 6	Del	
4 8	Amb	
5 20	D	
6 9	R	
7 4	L	
8 21	R	
9 17	Del	
10 3	D	
11 12	Amb	
12 23	D	
13 10	L	
14 11	Del	
15 19	D	
16 14	R	
17 13	R	
18 2	Amb	
19 15	L	
20 16	Amb	
21 22	Del	
22 7	L	
23 24	R	
24 25	Del	
25 18	L	

TOTAL MATCHES BY CATEGORY FORM

Question Number*	Decisions**	Question Number	Risk	Question Number	Ambiguity	Question Number	Delegating	Question Number	Lifestyle
1		6		2		3		7	
5		8		4		9		13	
10		16		11		14		19	
12		17		18		21		22	
15		23		20		24		25	
Totals by Category		Totals by Category		Totals by Category		Totals by Category		Totals by Category	
% Match		% Match		% Match		% Match		% Match	

Total Score: _____

Total Percentage: _____

* Numbers match questions on the "Self Assessment Checklist."
** Transfer check marks from "Score By Question Form" which matches corresponding items from the "Self Assessment" and "Job Assessment" Checklists.

Timothy H. Lentner, MSW, is currently Program Administrator of the Adult Services and Medical/Health Service programs of Washtenaw County Community Mental Health in Ann Arbor, Michigan. He is a past board member of the National Council of Community Mental Health Centers and a past president of the National Association for Rural Mental Health (NARMH). He served as an evaluator of the NIMH-funded Rural Mental Health Demonstration Projects in 1989-1990. He is a frequent presenter at NARMH's annual conference. Mr. Lentner may be contacted at Washtenaw County Community Mental Health, 2140 E. Ellsworth, Box 8645, Ann Arbor, MI 48107.

Saul Cooper, MA, is currently Director of the Human Services Department of Washtenaw County and Adjunct Professor of Psychology and Psychiatry at the University of Michigan, Ann Arbor. He was the Washtenaw County Administrator from 1987 to 1991 and Director of the Washtenaw County Community Mental Health Center. He is an Editorial Advisory Board member of the *Community Mental Health Journal*, the *Journal of Consultation*, and the *Journal of Prevention*. Mr. Cooper can be contacted at Washtenaw County, Human Services Department, P.O. Box 915, Ypsilanti, MI 48197-0915.

REFERENCES

Adia Personnel Services (ADIA). (1989). *News from Adia.* Menlo Park, CA: Author. (Adia is a national employment service which surveys potential employers about the dynamics of job placement.)

Fritz, R. (1980). Measuring managerial performance. *Small Business Report, March,* 18-20.

Jackson, S. E. (1983). Participation in decision making as a strategy for reducing job-related strain. *Journal of Applied Psychology, 68,* 3-19.

Jung, C. G. (1959). The self. In Sir H. Read, M. Fordham, & G. Adler (Eds.), *The Collected Works of C. G. Jung* (Bollingen Series, XX, Vol. 9, Part II, Chapter 4, p. 23 ff). New York: Pantheon Books.

Locke, E. (1988, August 15). Powerful motivators, part one: Money, money, money. *Practical Supervision, N. 76,* 1-2.

Mintzberg, H. (1975). The manager's job: Folklore and fact. *Harvard Business Review, 53,* 49-61.

Moos, R. H. (1974a). *Evaluating Correctional and Community Settings.* New York: John Wiley & Sons.

Moos, R. H. (1974b). *Evaluating Treatment Environments.* New York: John Wiley & Sons.

10

Community Mental Health in the Year 2000*

*James W. Stockdill, Loretta K. Haggard,
and Robin L. Michaelson*

The public mental health system has been described as a "nonsystem" that is inaccessible, fragmented, and incomplete (General Accounting Office, 1977; Talbott, 1978, 1987). In too many communities, mental health care is splintered between institutional and community programs, and between the public and private sectors. Mental health treatment, housing, and supports (including educational and vocational services, health care, substance abuse treatment, and entitlement programs), to the extent they are available to mentally ill persons, are provided by diverse agencies, each with different eligibility requirements and application procedures. Because of these limitations and resource constraints, many patients are forced into costly and inappropriate treatment, unnecessary confinement (e.g., jails), or receive no care at all. To modify the present patchwork of care so that it is more responsive to the multiple and changing needs of severely mentally ill individuals, there will need to be extensive changes in the infrastructure underlying mental health care (Levine, Lezak, & Goldman, 1986; Morrissey & Goldman, 1984).

This challenge is even more difficult than it may seem upon first glance. The long-term, severely mentally ill population served by community mental health programs and state mental hospitals is both growing in number and becoming more hetero-

*The opinions expressed herein are those of the authors and do not necessarily reflect the official policy of the National Institute of Mental Health. The authors would like to thank Irene S. Levine, PhD, for her editorial suggestions and comments.

213

geneous. There may be as many as 4 million individuals with severe mental illness in the United States (National Institute of Mental Health, 1992). Among the most rapidly growing subgroups of the severely mentally ill population are the elderly, children and adolescents, minorities, dually diagnosed persons, and homeless persons. The number of severely mentally ill persons who are living with AIDS is also growing. Given this diversity, most community mental health programs will require special adaptations to serve the specialized needs of these subgroups.

This chapter first briefly defines long-term severe mental illness and describes efforts of the National Institute of Mental Health (NIMH) to assist states and localities in developing appropriate services for the population. It identifies several subgroups of the severely mentally ill population, describes their current service needs, and projects their future needs. It then describes the organizational and financing reforms that will be required in the existing mental health system to meet the needs of the severely mentally ill population in the year 2000. The chapter is not intended to be exhaustive; the references cited can provide a more in-depth analysis of issues that are just touched upon here.

THE SEVERELY MENTALLY ILL POPULATION

Individuals with long-term mental illnesses have variously been labeled chronically mentally ill, seriously mentally ill, or, more recently, severely mentally ill. This target population is generally defined by the dimensions of diagnosis, disability, and duration (Bachrach, 1988; Goldman, Gattozzi, & Taube, 1981). These individuals suffer from major mental disorders (such as schizophrenia, schizoaffective disorders, mood disorders, or severe personality disorders), are functionally incapacitated by their illnesses, and have either persistent or recurrent long-term disabilities (Goldman et al., 1981).

Since 1977, the NIMH Community Support Program (CSP) has focused its efforts on this target population and has awarded grants to states to improve local community support systems. The program is premised on meeting the interrelated mental health and social welfare needs of severely mentally ill individuals (Stroul, 1984; Turner & Shifren, 1979; Turner & TenHoor, 1978), an approach that departs from prior efforts to assist this population in the community (Levine et al., 1986; Morrissey &

Goldman, 1984). The CSP program has also supported systems-improvement projects to assist state mental health agencies, as well as demonstration projects focusing on various subgroups of the target population. More recently, CSP has supported research demonstration projects to test and evaluate the effectiveness of innovative interventions such as psychosocial rehabilitation, case management, and crisis intervention.

THE ELDERLY

As many as 15% to 25% of persons aged 65 and older have significant mental health problems (U.S. Senate Special Committee on Aging, 1991). Approximately 4% to 7% of elderly Americans suffer from severe dementia, and an additional 5% to 8% suffer from moderate to mild dementia (Lebowitz & Cohen, 1992). Major depressive disorders, phobias, dysphoria, polydrug use and abuse, and alcohol abuse also are prevalent among this subgroup (Action Committee, 1986). These psychiatric problems are often compounded by the isolation, health problems, and financial stressors that accompany aging (Action Committee, 1986).

Financial problems (e.g., inadequate Medicaid, Medicare, and third-party insurance coverage), transportation barriers, and difficulties in identifying and accessing services too often pose formidable obstacles for elderly mentally ill persons who might want to avail themselves of mental health care. Although more than 600 community mental health centers (CMHCs) see increasing numbers of elderly mentally ill individuals, only half of the CMHCs have services designed specifically for the elderly mentally ill population. In addition, there is a paucity of clinical staff with geriatric expertise (Lebowitz, 1988).

Assertive case management is essential to link these individuals to appropriate services and entitlement programs. An ideal service system for elderly mentally ill individuals would provide care in a variety of settings, including the community, nursing homes, and hospitals for institutional care, and would include community-based services such as activity centers, day care, congregate meals, assisted housing, home health care, and respite care (Lebowitz, in press). Because of physical infirmities and the emotional insecurities that accompany the aging process, many elderly mentally ill persons require transportation to take advantage of community mental health services and appropriate day treatment programs.

ween 1980 and 2000, the U.S. population between the
65 and 74 can be expected to increase by 17%, and the
ion over age 85 will double (U.S. Senate Special Commit-
Aging, 1991). These demographic trends will require
tention to the needs of elderly mentally ill individuals in
r 2000. Outreach to private homes, nursing homes, area
s for the aging (AAA), and senior citizen centers can
identifying, locating, and engaging this subgroup into
(Action Committee, 1986). In a number of communities,
aboration of CMHCs and AAAs increases the effective-
the mental health program (Lebowitz, 1988).

CHILDREN AND ADOLESCENTS

More than 12% of the U.S. population aged 18 and under, or
7.5 million young Americans, may need mental health services,
and 3 million children and adolescents may be considered severely emotionally disturbed (National Advisory Mental Health
Council, 1990). Mental health problems of children and adolescents result from interactions between individual vulnerabilities
and environmental risk factors. Factors that place children at risk
for severe emotional or mental disorder include failure to receive
basic nurturance, mental illness in the family, child abuse or
neglect, chronic physical illness, substance abuse, homelessness,
and other environmental stressors.

Funding for mental health services for children has been
decidedly inadequate (Dougherty, 1988). Less than one-fifth of
emotionally disturbed children and adolescents receive appropriate care (National Advisory Mental Health Council, 1990).
Moreover, the limited treatment resources available often have
been used to remove severely emotionally disturbed children and
adolescents from their families and place them (often unneces-
sarily) for long periods of time in restrictive living environments
(Friesen et al., 1988). Treatment for mental health disorders in
young Americans costs more than $1.5 billion annually (National
Advisory Mental Health Council, 1990).

The NIMH Child and Adolescent Service System Program
(CASSP) emphasizes the importance of comprehensive services
that are oriented toward both the child and his or her family
(Lourie & Katz-Leavy, 1987). The services needed by severely
emotionally disturbed children and adolescents cut across multiple service systems and include: residential and nonresidential
mental health services (e.g., early intervention, crisis interven-

tion, home-based services, day treatment, and therapeutic foster care); social services (e.g., home services and respite care); educational services (e.g., special education and homebound instruction); and "operational services" (e.g., case management, self-help, and transportation). Treatments vary according to the nature of specific childhood disorders and environmental factors (Saxe, Cross, & Silverman, 1988).

Based upon the recommendations of the *National Plan for Research on Child and Adolescent Mental Disorders* (National Advisory Mental Health Council, 1990), NIMH funds research demonstrations of innovative service system models that follow principles of multiagency, community-based, child- and family-centered care. These programs must be culturally sensitive and include families in assessment, planning, and implementation. In addition, legislation has recently been introduced in Congress to provide grants for child mental health services.

MINORITIES

By the year 2000, members of racial and ethnic minority groups - which include African-Americans, Asians, Hispanics, and Native Americans - will comprise a substantial proportion of the U.S. population. Although prevalence rates of mental illness are higher among minorities than among whites, these rates are confounded by low socioeconomic status, which is also correlated with a higher prevalence of mental health problems (Robins & Regier, 1991).

In addition to problems of availability and access, language barriers, immigration status, or prior negative experiences with the mental health or social services system may make minority persons who would otherwise benefit from community mental health care reluctant to seek out formal, structured programs. Therefore, outreach and other informal means of engagement are necessary and might most appropriately take place in the client's home or some other familiar setting (Toff & Welch, 1988). Minority persons who are severely mentally ill need therapists, case managers, and outreach workers who understand the cultural background and language of their clients (Task Force, 1992). Because of the socioeconomic problems often experienced by minority persons, clinicians must assist clients in meeting their basic needs. Advocacy and empowerment are especially critical in the therapeutic process with members of minority groups who may have previously met with discrimination and economic hardship (Grevious, 1985).

DUALLY DIAGNOSED PERSONS

Persons with co-occurring mental illness and alcohol and/or other drug abuse problems also present a great challenge to the mental health system. In many areas of the country, dual diagnosis is more often the rule, rather than the exception, among persons seeking care at mental health agencies. At least one-half of the homeless severely mentally ill population abuse alcohol and/or drugs (Task Force, 1992).

The dually diagnosed severely mentally ill population is generally characterized by polydrug use and abuse, with substances of choice including alcohol, marijuana, LSD, amphetamines, PCP, cocaine, Quaaludes, glue, and barbiturates (Safer, 1986). On average, the rates of use of these substances among mentally ill persons are three times greater than those of high school seniors, college students, or medical outpatients (Safer, 1986). Even minimal use of drugs and/or alcohol can be destabilizing for a person with severe mental illness (Drake, Osher, & Wallach, 1989).

One of the challenges of working with this population is in assessing the patient's condition and ascertaining the relative contributions of mental illness and substance abuse to the patient's presenting problems (Ridgely, Osher, & Talbott, 1987). Treatment is also difficult because most clinicians are trained in only one field (mental health or substance abuse) and have little understanding of the other orientation. Because of such problems, these patients are frequently shuttled back and forth between programs; when they are accepted in a program, treatment may actually conflict with their best interests. For example, a rule of abstinence (from all psychoactive substances) in a residential program for substance abusers may conflict with a severely mentally ill patient's need for prescribed psychotropic medication.

Both assessment and treatment of these patients must be comprehensive and sensitive to the interactions of the two disorders. A proper treatment program would address this population's tendency to overutilize inappropriate, more intensive services like hospital emergency rooms; it would include medication management, individual and group counseling, crisis intervention, social support, residential and vocational assistance, case management, family support and education, detoxification, drug education, peer support, and self-help groups (Ridgely et al., 1987). Expectations regarding the outcomes of treatment must be realistic, given the multiple disabilities and often cyclical nature of mental illness and substance abuse problems (Ridgely et al., 1987).

HOMELESS MENTALLY ILL PERSONS

Because of definitional ambiguities and methodological challenges, it is difficult to make reliable estimates of the exact numbers of persons who are homeless and mentally ill (Levine & Haggard, 1989; Levine & Rog, 1990). A General Accounting Office report (1988) acknowledged in its review of 27 national, state, and local studies that there were no sound national estimates of the size of the homeless population. Recently, there has been considerable debate over the shelter and street count conducted by the Census Bureau in its 1990 decennial census. Definitions of homelessness vary widely from study to study and encompass a range of variables such as lack of shelter, income, social support, or affiliation with others.

The homeless population includes adults, children and their families, the elderly, the dually diagnosed, and persons with AIDS. Minority populations comprise a substantial proportion of all these subgroups. The Federal Task Force on Homelessness and Severe Mental Illness (1992) estimates that there may be up to 600,000 persons nationally who are homeless on a given day.

NIMH-supported research studies suggest that approximately one-third of the homeless single adult population suffer from a severe mental illness (Levine & Rog, 1990; Tessler & Dennis, 1989). The studies also shed light on the special characteristics and needs of this subgroup. For example, homeless mentally ill persons generally need help in multiple areas, such as alcohol and/or other drug abuse problems, acute or chronic health problems, and vocational and social deficits. Because of their histories of residential instability, homeless mentally ill persons tend to have few housing options open to them. A surprisingly large proportion of the target group is or has been involved with the criminal justice system (NIMH, 1991).

In 1987, the Stewart B. McKinney Homeless Assistance Act (Public Law 100-77, as amended by Public Law 100-628 and Public Law 101-645) outlined a range of comprehensive mental health and support services necessary to address the needs of this subgroup: outreach to shelters and streets and other places where homeless mentally ill people can be found; intensive case management that focuses on meeting clients' subsistence and mental health treatment needs; mental health treatment that is flexible, accessible, and nonthreatening; and a continuum of residential services from emergency shelters and drop-in centers, to transitional residences, to permanent independent or supported housing. Current NIMH McKinney research demonstrations and a formula grant program to the states now focus on providing comprehensive community mental health services coordinated with housing services to homeless mentally ill individuals.

Homeless mentally ill individuals are often disenfranchised both from programs designed for mentally ill persons and programs designed for the homeless population (Levine, 1984). To work with this population, a great deal of time and effort must be made to "engage" the population in services and to provide services in flexible, nontraditional ways (Rog, 1988). The needs of the homeless dually diagnosed population require coordination between the mental health and substance abuse treatment systems (Drake, Osher, & Wallach, 1991).

AIDS

At least 1 million Americans currently are infected with the HIV virus that causes Acquired Immunodeficiency Syndrome (National Commission on Acquired Immune Deficiency Syndrome, 1991). Little definitive information is available on the prevalence of HIV infection among mentally ill individuals, but preliminary data suggests that seroprevalence rates are elevated among this group compared to the general population. HIV infection rates appear higher among the homeless mentally ill population.

Some mentally ill individuals engage in behaviors that increase their risk of AIDS. Despite stereotypes of asexuality, mentally ill persons (like others of their age cohort) are sexually active, and some, associated with their mental illness, may impulsively pursue sexual activity, both homosexual and heterosexual (Carmen & Brady, 1990). The high incidence of substance use and abuse among the mentally ill population, and particularly the homeless mentally ill population, also increases their risk of contracting AIDS through intravenous drug use and behavioral disinhibition.

AIDS education and prevention efforts need to be modified to be effective for the mentally ill population. Mentally ill persons may have less access to knowledge about how to avoid health risks and fewer resources for health maintenance and prevention. Impaired judgment or concentration may complicate attempts to educate a mentally ill individual about effective interventions, such as safe sex or the use of clean needles. Modifications may also need to be made in approaches to treating HIV infections, particularly among the homeless mentally ill population who may not have access to long-term health care.

ESSENTIAL QUALITIES OF THE
COMMUNITY MENTAL HEALTH CARE SYSTEM
IN THE YEAR 2000

Clearly, the changing composition of the severely mentally ill population will necessitate major reforms in community mental health care. Based upon our discussion of subpopulations and their needs, we anticipate that the following qualities will be essential to the community mental health system in the year 2000:

1. *Given*: The severely mentally ill population is heterogeneous, and includes elderly persons, children and adolescents, minorities, dually diagnosed persons, homeless persons, and persons with AIDS.
   Implications: Special adaptations in community mental health programming will be required to care for these diverse subgroups. Of course, these adaptations will necessitate increased specialization in both academic and inservice training of mental health professionals.
2. *Given*: Most persons with long-term, severe mental illness have comprehensive service needs extending far beyond mental health treatment alone.
   Implications: Community mental health programs will increasingly need to provide comprehensive programming, focusing not just on clients' mental health needs, but also on housing, income, health, vocational, educational, and social needs. Rather than providing an office-based model limited to traditional clinical care, community mental health programs need to make assertive clinical case management services available to assist severely mentally ill persons in gaining access to the wide range of programs that can meet their needs. This will necessitate improved

linkages at both the client and the service system levels and between agencies, and training opportunities crossing over multiple disciplines (e.g., mental illness and substance abuse, mental illness and aging).

3. *Given*: Many severely mentally ill individuals are willing to accept assistance but are unable, because of their disabilities or other barriers, to seek help on their own from the traditional mental health system.

   Implications: Rather than waiting for severely mentally ill persons to seek help themselves, community mental health providers will need to be more assertive and provide outreach in the community. In the case of homeless persons this will require the availability of services in shelters, soup kitchens, or on the streets. Many elderly mentally ill persons who could or would not seek assistance on their own may be receptive to assistance offered at the local senior citizen's center.

4. *Given*: The needs of severely mentally ill persons are dynamic and change over time.

   Implications: A rigid model of community mental health care, whereby clients "graduate" from one level and type of care to another and then from the system altogether is inappropriate for many severely mentally ill persons. Insofar as the community mental health system shifts its focus toward this client population, then it must shift its emphasis and expectations; care, not cure, must become the aim. A range of intensities of residential options, treatment, and supervision is more appropriate than a continuum of care, which focuses on moving clients through and out of the system. Ongoing needs assessment and continuous case management will be essential features of the community mental health system.

THE STRUCTURE OF THE PUBLICLY FUNDED COMMUNITY MENTAL HEALTH SYSTEM

The organization and financing of the current system is poorly suited to meet the heterogeneous and changing needs of severely mentally ill individuals. Reimbursement for mental health care is often limited to office-based medical-model treatment, rather than nontraditional outreach and assertive case management focusing on clients' multiple needs. In addition, because case managers generally do not have the ability to purchase appropriate services for their clients, case managers tend to lack effectiveness in service planning.

Our discussion of the community-based mental health system of the future is predicated on at least two assumptions:

1. All states, with federal encouragement and funding support, will have established the most severely disabled mentally ill population as the highest priority for public mental health services; and
2. The programmatic focus of most community mental health centers will be consistent with state policies and priorities.

To meet the multiple, diverse, and long-term needs of the severely mentally ill population, the community service system in the year 2000 will need to be restructured so that local financing and management entities receive funds on a prepaid capitated basis. These local systems management entities could be community mental health centers, city or county departments of mental health, or new authorities specifically developed and authorized by the state to manage and fund services. The local entities would be responsible for serving all severely mentally ill individuals in their service area and would have a unified budget to fund the wide range of services needed by the population.

Capitation financing is generally defined as prospective payments to providers on a per person basis for a predetermined set of services. A capitation approach would require a clear definition of the priority population and the establishment of population-based needs assessment procedures. A capitated system would provide incentives for a coordinated set of essential services that can reduce the costs of long-term inpatient care; this managed system would also provide incentives and opportunities to reallocate resources from large institutions to community-based care (Vischi & Stockdill, 1988).

Capitation financing would provide incentives to effectively plan, organize, and manage individualized services appropriate for the severely mentally ill population and would also control costs. Allocation of funds to service providers would be based on contemporary performance contracting principles (Stockdill, 1987). The entities would be directed by individuals trained in systems development with good management skills. A systems-wide management information system would assure adequate data for needs assessment and program planning, treatment and rehabilitation planning, client tracking, and program evaluation.

Case managers, employed directly by the entities, would coordinate services from the perspective of individual clients; case managers would help clients access and utilize the system developed by the systems managers. They also would provide effective accountability and evaluation mechanisms to assure that the system is working. Each case manager would have to understand the range of service needs, available services, and financing mechanisms.

The local authority would provide a single point of entry into the system with mechanisms in place for preadmission screening to inpatient care and joint discharge planning. Mechanisms for quality assurance would include program and staffing standards, and staff development and training in treatment, rehabilitation, and management skills. An independent community protection and advocacy entity would assure the protection of client rights and the investigation of grievances and allegations of abuse and neglect. There would be a variety of mechanisms for consumer, family, and citizen input into program planning, management, and evaluation.

FINANCING OF THE COMMUNITY SERVICE SYSTEM

Funds for the proposed prepaid capitated community mental health system would come mainly from state and federal financing mechanisms. For the severely mentally ill population under age 65, this would necessitate changes in the Medicaid program that would make funds available through the states to the local authorities on a flexible basis to support a package of community support services (Vischi & Stockdill, 1988). Additional state revenues would be needed to fund the planning, management, and evaluative functions of the local authorities. In most states, localities would have to match these state funds for systems management. Decreases in the utilization of state hospitals could make additional state revenues available for both the Medicaid funding program and the funding of local authority governance responsibilities. For the severely mentally ill population over age 65, there would need to be a new federally subsidized long-term care group insurance program, emphasizing home health care, social support, and respite care (Hastings, 1986).

These projected federal and state financing trends and policies might well result in what would be seen as a dual system of care - with the publicly funded system serving the needs of the long-term severely mentally ill population, and those persons with acute mental health problems being served by private practitioners and the general health care system (Larsen, 1986). Community mental health centers and other local vendors within the publicly funded managed mental health care system would have the option of serving acutely mentally ill populations through private sector financing. As they did, however, they would find themselves in increasing competition with the private for-profit health care sector. However, there also might be incentives to encourage private mental health practitioners to spend a significant portion of their time working with clients of the public mental health system (Sharfstein & Beigel, 1988). This would help provide important coordinating links between the two systems.

MANAGED CARE

Throughout the 1980s, private insurers have been applying "managed care" approaches to the utilization of mental health benefits under insurance plans. Largely developed in the health care field, these approaches are generally directed at controlling costs through assuring appropriate utilization of services. The many forms of managed care make defining the term difficult (Dorwart, 1990). Nevertheless, since the late 1980s these same approaches are increasingly being applied to the management of publicly funded services under the Medicaid program and state general revenues.

The developing application of managed care approaches to publicly funded mental health services usually comes through contracts with private management organizations which frequently offer the following general services: development and management of capitated funding approaches; utilization review of mental health outpatient and inpatient services; quality assurance programs; case management for high utilizers of services; and outcome assessment activities.

Intrusion into the patient-doctor relationship and related violations of privacy and confidentiality are the most frequently cited negative impact of managed care services (Borenstein, 1990). These problems in turn may affect continuity and quality of care. A positive aspect of managed care is that utilization management assists in the achievement of a more rational mental health service system. Inappropriate utilizations can be reduced, costs controlled, and third party funding benefits protected and expanded. As Patterson (1990) has indicated, a managed care system able to construct the right delivery model, select the appropriate providers, employ judicious financial incentives, and undertake adequate oversight will achieve rational mental health care delivery.

Currently, managed care of mental health benefits remains a panacea to some and an anathema to others. However, it seems clear that the lessons learned from the managed care applications of the early 1990s will determine the extent of successful implementation of the structural and funding changes in the community mental health system. In addition, the development of a national health insurance program with mental health benefits is again part of the national health funding debate (Weil, 1991). The lessons learned from managed care applications may well help determine the equitable coverage for services to the mentally ill population under any national health care program.

CONCLUSIONS

Although no one can predict the future with certainty, understanding the present is the most reliable way to anticipate the future (Naisbitt, 1982). It is evident that the pervasive problems experienced by severely mentally ill individuals and their families in accessing and receiving comprehensive community-based care will demand a major restructuring of the service system by or before the year 2000. Such a change must, of course, be predicated upon a thorough understanding of the complex and interrelated changing treatment and support needs of severely mentally ill persons. Restructuring the system in an era of fiscal retrenchment and resource constraints will also require creative innovations in the organization and financing of community mental health care. Hopefully we will rise to these daunting challenges through improved knowledge in the areas of treatment and services (based on research and demonstration efforts) and strategic planning, and through a tenacious commitment to improved services for long-term, severely mentally ill persons.

James W. Stockdill, MA, is currently Deputy Director
of the Maryland Mental Hygiene Administration.
Prior to this position, he served for over 20 years with
the National Institute of Mental Health in several
positions concerned with the planning and evaluation
of mental health services, research, and training programs. His major interest is in the analysis of federal,
state, and local roles and responsibilities in the delivery and financing of mental health services. Mr.
Stockdill may be contacted at Mental Hygiene Administration, 201 West Preston Street, 4th Floor, Baltimore, MD 21201.

Loretta K. Haggard is presently working on a joint
JD/MSW degree at Washington University in St.
Louis. Prior to this she was a case manager at CASA
Homeless Service Program in St. Louis and was the
Assistant Coordinator for the National Institute of
Mental Health Program for the Homeless Mentally Ill.
She received her Bachelor of Arts degree from Prince-
ton. Ms. Haggard can be contacted at 5041 Waterman
Boulevard, St. Louis, MO 63108.

Robin L. Michaelson, MSc, is currently a public health
analyst in the National Institute of Mental Health Office of Programs for the Homeless Mentally Ill. She
received her Masters in Public Policy from the London
School of Economics and her Bachelor of Arts degree
from Princeton. Ms. Michaelson can be contacted at
the Office of Programs for the Homeless Mentally Ill,
National Institute of Mental Health, 5600 Fishers
Lane, Room 7C-08, Rockville, MD 20857.

REFERENCES

Action Committee to Implement the Mental Health Recommendations of the 1981 White House Conference on Aging.
(1986). *Report on a Survey of Community Mental Health
Centers* (Vol. III). Washington, DC: Author.
Bachrach, L. L. (1988). Defining chronic mental illness: A
concept paper. *Hospital and Community Psychiatry, 39,* 383-
388.

Borenstein, D. B. (1990). Managed care: A means of rationing psychiatric treatment. *Hospital and Community Psychiatry, 41,* 10.

Carmen, E., & Brady, S. (1990, June). AIDS risk and prevention for the chronically mentally ill. *Hospital and Community Psychiatry, 41,* 652-657.

Dorwart, R. A. (1990). Managed mental health care: Myths and realities in the 1990s. *Hospital and Community Psychiatry, 41,* 10.

Dougherty, D. (1988). Children's mental health problems and services: Current federal efforts and policy implications. *American Psychologist, 43,* 808.

Drake, R. E., Osher, F. C., & Wallach, M. A. (1989). Alcohol use and abuse in schizophrenia: A prospective community study. *Journal of Nervous and Mental Disease, 177,* 408-414.

Drake, R. E., Osher, F. C., & Wallach, M. A. (1991, November). Homelessness and dual diagnosis. *American Psychologist, 46,* 1149-1158.

Friesen, B. J., Griesbach, J., Jacobs, J. H., Katz-Leavy, J., & Olson, D. (1988). Improving services for families. *Children Today, 17,* 18.

General Accounting Office. (1977). *Returning the Mentally Disabled to the Community: Government Needs to do More* (Publication No. HRD-76-152). Washington, DC: U.S. Government Printing Office.

General Accounting Office. (1988). *Homeless Mentally Ill: Problems and Options in Estimating Numbers and Trends.* A U.S. General Accounting Office Report to the Chairman, Committee on Labor and Human Resources, U.S. Senate, Washington, DC.

Goldman, H. H., Gattozzi, A. A., & Taube, C. A. (1981). Defining and counting the chronically mentally ill. *Hospital and Community Psychiatry, 32,* 21-27.

Grevious, C. (1985). The role of the family therapist with low-income black families. *Family Therapy, 12,* 115-122.

Hastings, M. M. (1986). The long-term care puzzle and mental health policy: Putting the pieces together. *American Behavioral Scientist, 30,* 143-174.

Larsen, J. K. (1986). Local mental health agencies in transition. *American Behavioral Scientist, 30,* 174-187.

Lebowitz, B. D. (1988). Mental health policy & aging. *Generations: Public Policy,* pp. 53-56.

Lebowitz, B. D. (in press). Community services for the elderly psychiatric patient. In H. I. Kaplan & B. J. Sadock (Eds.),

Comprehensive Textbook of Psychiatry (6th ed.). Baltimore, MD: Williams & Wilkins.

Lebowitz, B. D., & Cohen, G. S. (1992). The elderly and their illness. In C. Salzman (Ed.), *Clinical Geriatric Psychopharmacology* (2nd ed.). Baltimore, MD: Williams & Wilkins.

Levine, I. S. (1984). Service programs for the homeless mentally ill. In H. R. Lamb (Ed.), *The Homeless Mentally Ill* (pp. 173-200). Washington, DC: American Psychiatric Association.

Levine, I. S., & Haggard, L. K. (1989). Homelessness as a public mental health problem. In D. A. Rochefort (Ed.), *Handbook on Mental Health Policy in the United States* (pp. 293-310). Boston: Greenwood Press.

Levine, I. S., Lezak, A. D., & Goldman, H. H. (1986). Community support systems for the homeless mentally ill. In E. L. Bassuk (Ed.), *The Mental Health Needs of Homeless Persons* (New Directions for Mental Health Services, p. 30). San Francisco: Jossey-Bass.

Levine, I. S., & Rog, D. J. (1990). Mental health services for homeless mentally ill persons: Federal initiatives and current service trends. *American Psychologist, 45,* 963-968.

Lourie, I. S., & Katz-Leavy, J. (1987). Severely emotionally disturbed children and adolescents. In W. W. Menninger & G. Hannah (Eds.), *The Chronic Mental Patient II* (pp. 159-185). Washington, DC: American Psychiatric Press.

Morrissey, J. P., & Dennis, D. L. (1986). *NIMH-Funded Research Concerning Homeless Mentally Ill Persons: Implications for Policy and Practice.* Rockville, MD: National Institute of Mental Health.

Morrissey, J. P., & Goldman, H. H. (1984). Cycles of reform in the care of the chronically mentally ill. *Hospital and Community Psychiatry, 35,* 785-793.

Naisbitt, J. (1982). *Megatrends: Ten New Directions Transforming Our Lives.* New York: Warner Books.

National Advisory Mental Health Council. (1990). *A National Plan for Research on Child and Adolescent Mental Disorders.* Rockville, MD: National Institute of Mental Health.

National Commission on Acquired Immune Deficiency Syndrome. (1991). *America Living with AIDS.* Washington, DC: U.S. Government Printing Office.

National Institute of Mental Health. (1991). *Two Generations of NIMH-Funded Research on Homelessness and Mental Illness: 1982-1990.* Rockville, MD: Author.

National Institute of Mental Health, Statistical Research Branch. (1992). Unpublished estimate.

Patterson, D. Y. (1990). Managed care: An approach to rational psychiatric treatment. *Hospital and Community Psychiatry, 41*, 10.

Ridgely, M. S., Goldman, H. H., & Talbott, J. A. (1986). *Chronic Mentally Ill Young Adults with Substance Abuse Problems: A Review of Relevant Literature and Creation of a Research Agenda.* Baltimore, MD: University of Maryland Task Force on Chronic Mentally Ill Young Adults with Substance Abuse Problems.

Ridgely, M. S., Osher, F. C., & Talbott, J. A. (1987). *Chronic Mentally Ill Young Adults with Substance Abuse Problems. Treatment and Training Issues.* Baltimore, MD: University of Maryland Task Force on Chronic Mentally Ill Young Adults with Substance Abuse Problems.

Robins, L. N., & Regier, D. A. (Eds.). (1991). *Psychiatric Disorders in America: The Epidemiologic Catchment Area Study.* New York: Macmillan.

Rog, D. J. (1988). *Engaging Homeless Persons with Mental Illness into Treatment.* Rockville, MD: National Institute of Mental Health.

Safer, D. (1986). The young adult chronic patient and substance use disorders: Description and rationale. *American Journal of Psychiatry, 143*, 463-468. (Cited in Ridgely et al., 1986, p. 24.)

Saxe, L., Cross, T., & Silverman, N. (1988). Children's mental health: The gap between what we know and what we do. *American Psychologist, 43*, 800-807.

Schuster, C. R. (1988). A federal agency perspective on AIDS. *American Psychologist, 43*, 846.

Sharfstein, S. S., & Beigel, A. (1988). How to service in the private practice of psychiatry. *American Journal of Psychiatry, 145*, 723-727.

Stockdill, J. W. (1987). *Financing Issues. Toward a Model Plan for a Comprehensive Community-Based Mental Health System.* Rockville, MD: National Institute of Mental Health.

Stroul, B. A. (1984). *Toward Community Support Systems for the Mentally Disabled: The NIMH Community Support Program.* Submitted to National Institute of Mental Health, Office of State and Community Liaison, Community Support and Rehabilitation Branch, Boston University Center for Rehabilitation Research and Training in Mental Health.

Talbott, J. A. (Ed.). (1978). *The Chronic Mental Patient, Problems, Solutions, and Recommendations for a Public Policy.* Prepared by The Ad Hoc Committee on the Chronic Mental Patient, The American Psychiatric Association, Washington, DC.

Talbott, J. A. (1987). *The Chronic Mentally Ill: What Do We Now Know, and Why Aren't We Implementing What We Know.* In W. W. Menninger & G. Hannah (Eds.), *The Chronic Mental Patient II* (pp. 1-129). Washington, DC: American Psychiatric Press.

Task Force on Homelessness and Severe Mental Illness. (1992). *Outcasts on Main Street: Report of the Federal Task Force on Homelessness and Severe Mental Illness.* Washington, DC: Author.

Tessler, R. C., & Dennis, D. L. (1989). *A Synthesis of NIMH-Funded Research Concerning Persons Who Are Homeless and Mentally Ill.* Rockville, MD: National Institute of Mental Health.

Toff, G., & Welch, W. M. (1988). *Service Needs of Homeless and Homeless Mentally Ill Minority Persons.* Rockville, MD: National Institute of Mental Health.

Tross, S., & Hirsch, D. A. (1988). Psychological distress and neuropsychological complications of HIV infection and AIDS. *American Psychologist, 43,* 929.

Turner, J. C., & Shifren, I. (1979). Community support systems: How comprehensive? In H. R. Lamb (Ed.), *New Directions for Mental Health Services* (Vol. 2, pp. 1-13). San Francisco: Jossey-Bass.

Turner, J. C., & TenHoor, W. (1978). The NIMH community support program: Pilot approach to a needed social reform. *Schizophrenia Bulletin, 4,* 319-348.

U.S. Department of Health and Human Services. (1980). *Toward a National Plan for the Chronically Mentally Ill.* Washington, DC: Author.

U.S. Senate Special Committee on Aging, the American Association of Retired Persons, the Federal Council on the Aging, and the U.S. Administration on Aging. (1991). *Aging America: Trends and Projects.* Washington, DC: Author.

Vischi, T. R., & Stockdill, J. W. (1989). The financing of comprehensive community support systems: A review of major strategies. *Psychosocial Rehabilitation Journal, 12,* 83-92.

Weil, T. P. (1991). Mental health services under a U.S. national health insurance plan. *Hospital and Community Psychiatry, 42,* 7.

Index

Reagan administration, 128
Reagan, President, 6, 15
Records, 46, 69
Regier, D. A., 141, 217
Rehabilitation services, 8-10, 142
Reihman, J., 74
Research, 12, 156
    integration with practice, 149
Residential care services, 142, 220, 222
Resistance
    to community mental health
        organization growth, 63-64
    to treatment, 74
Resnick, Eugene, 19
Retardation, mental, 109, 115
Retrospective review programs, 26
Ridgely, M. S., 218, 219
Risk behaviors for AIDS, 220
Risk in community mental health
        centers, 28-29, 37-43
Risk management programs, 67-68, 69
Risk Retention Act, 58
Robinowitz, C. B., 16
Robins, L. N., 217
Rog, D. J., 219, 220
Rubin, A., 152
Rural communities, 114-115
    services in, 7
Ryglewicz, Hilary, 73, 74, 88, 89, 92

S

Safer, D., 218
Sagner, B., 117-118
Saxe, L., 217
Schizoaffective disorders, 214
Schizophrenia, 8, 79, 148, 154, 214
Schwartz, S., 74
Sciacca, K., 89
Screening
    by correctional staff, 113
    precommitment, 142
Seattle, 9
Sederer, L. I., 154
Self-help groups, 90-91, 219
Shakow, D., 148
Sharfstein, S. S., 15, 225
Shea, J. G., 58
Sheets, J. L., 74
Shepherd v. Dickson County
        Sheriff's Department, 99
Sherman, L., 111, 112
Shifren, I., 214

Shifren, L., 12-13
Shore, J., 146
Shore, J. H., 10, 13, 131
Short-term care, 141
Shortell, S. M., 164
Sibulkin, A., 28
Silverman, N., 217
Silverman, W. H., 156-157
Skill development, 154-157, 160
Smith, C. J., 6
Social Security disability, 129
Social skills training, 13
Social work
    degrees necessary, 152
    preservice training in, 150-152
Spaulding, W., 148
Special populations, community
        mental health center service
        to, 141-165
Spielberger, C. D., 149
Staff development
    assessment of resources, 158-163
    budget constraints on, 157-158
    evaluation of, 164-165
    implementation, 165
    needs, identification of, 158-163
    recruitment, 55, 65, 66, 70
    training, 10-11, 13, 141, 143-165
State hospital movement, 19th
        century, 126
Steadman, H. J., 120
Steffen, G., 24
Stein, L. I., 12
Steinwachs, D., 34
Stern, R., 142
Stewart B. McKinney Homeless
        Assistance Act, 219-220
Stockdill, James W., 213, 223, 224, 227
Stress, services for, 3, 88
Stressors
    of aging, 215
    of children and adolescents, 216
Stroul, B. A., 214
Substance Abusing Mentally Ill
        (SAMI), 76
Substance use/abuse, 5, 6, 23, 24,
        27-28, 35-36, 53, 65, 73-92,
        109, 112, 129, 218-219, 220
    alcohol, 5, 6, 73-92, 218, 219
    among adolescents, 36, 216
    among children, 216
    among elderly, 215
    amphetamines, 76, 218

University of Houston, 148
University of Nebraska-Lincoln, 148
Urban programs, 7
U.S. Senate Special Committee on
    Aging, 215, 216
Utilization review, 26, 27, 32, 33, 34-35
Utilization Review Organizations
    (UROs), 29-30

V

Vaccaro, J., 130, 146
Valdiserri, E., 99
Veterans' Administration, 17, 147
Veterans, Vietnam, 14
Violence, 74
Vischi, T. R., 223, 224
Vocational programs, 61, 86, 88
Voluntary Hospitals of America, 57

W

Wallace, C., 23
Wallach, M. A., 218, 220
Washington, 9
Wasserman, D. B., 157
Weil, T. P., 226
Weiner-Pomerantz, R., 157
Welch, W. M., 217
Welfare, 129
Wheeler, J., 25
Wickizer, T., 25
Winslow, W., 146
Winslow, W. W., 16
Wisconsin, 12, 13
Women, services for, 14
Wood, J., 15
Woy, J. R., 157

Z

Zacker, J., 89

Some Of The Other Titles Available
From Professional Resource Press

Innovations in Clinical Practice: A Source Book - **11 Volumes**
    Hardbound edition (Vols. 3-11 only) per volume... $54.20
    Looseleaf binder edition (Vols. 1-11) per volume.. $59.20
Cognitive Therapy with Couples.. $17.70
Maximizing Third-Party Reimbursement in Your Mental Health Practice................. $32.70
Who Speaks for the Children?
    The Handbook of Individual and Class Child Advocacy.. $38.70
Post-Traumatic Stress Disorder:
    Assessment, Differential Diagnosis, and Forensic Evaluation............................. $27.70
Clinical Evaluations of School-Aged Children: A Structured Approach to
    the Diagnosis of Child and Adolescent Mental Disorders.................................... $22.70
Stress Management Training: A Group Leader's Guide... $14.70
Stress Management Workbook for Law Enforcement Officers.................................... $ 8.70
Fifty Ways to Avoid Malpractice:
    A Guidebook for Mental Health Professionals... $17.70
Keeping Up the Good Work:
    A Practitioner's Guide to Mental Health Ethics... $16.70
Think Straight! Feel Great! 21 Guides to Emotional Self-Control............................... $14.70
Computer-Assisted Psychological Evaluations:
    How to Create Testing Programs in BASIC... $22.70

Titles In Our Practitioner's Resource Series

Assessment and Treatment of Multiple Personality and Dissociative Disorders ● Clinical Guidelines for Involuntary Outpatient Treatment ● Cognitive Therapy for Personality Disorders: A Schema-Focused Approach ● Dealing with Anger Problems: Rational-Emotive Therapeutic Interventions ● Diagnosis and Treatment Selection for Anxiety Disorders ● Neuropsychological Evaluation of Head Injury ● Outpatient Treatment of Child Molesters ● Pathological Gambling: Conceptual, Diagnostic, and Treatment Issues ● Pre-Employment Screening for Psychopathology: A Guide to Professional Practice ● *Tarasoff* and Beyond: Legal and Clinical Considerations in the Treatment of Life-Endangering Patients ● Treating Adult Survivors of Childhood Sexual Abuse ● What Every Therapist Should Know about AIDS
All books in this series are $11.70 each

All prices include shipping charges. Foreign orders add $2.00 shipping to total. All orders from individuals and private institutions must be prepaid in full. Florida residents add 7%. Prices and availability subject to change without notice.

See Reverse Side For Ordering Information ⟶

To Order

To order by mail, please send name, address, and telephone number, along with check or credit card information (card number and expiration date) to:

Professional Resource Press
PO Box 15560
Sarasota, FL 34277-1560

For fastest service
(VISA/MasterCard/American Express/Discover orders only)
CALL 1-813-366-7913 or FAX 1-813-366-7971

Would You Like To Be
On Our Mailing List?

If so, please write, call, or fax the following information:

Name: _____

Address: _____

Address: _____

City/State/Zip: _____

Daytime Phone #: (_____) _____

To insure that we send you all appropriate mailings, please include your professional affiliation (e.g., psychologist, clinical social worker, marriage and family therapist, mental health counselor, school psychologist, psychiatrist, etc.).